MANUAL OF HAEMATOLOGY

Annabelle S.J. Baughan MRCP, MRCPath

Senior Registrar in Haematology, The Middlesex
Hospital Medical School and Central Middlesex
Hospital, UK

Andrew S.B. Hughes MA, MRCP, MRCPath

Consultant Pathologist, Royal Victoria
Hospital, Banjul, The Gambia; Visiting
Scientific Worker, Medical Research Council
Laboratories, Fajara, The Gambia

Keith G. Patterson MRCP, MRCPath

Consultant Haematologist, Redbridge District
Hospitals, UK

Louise Stirling MRCP, MRCPath

Senior Lecturer in Haematology, The London
Hospital, Whitechapel; Honorary Consultant
Haematologist, Newham District Hospital, UK

Churchill Livingstone

EDINBURGH LONDON MELBOURNE AND NEW YORK 1985

CHURCHILL LIVINGSTONE
Medical Division of Longman Group Limited

Distributed in the United States of America by
Churchill Livingstone Inc., 1560 Broadway, New York,
N.Y. 10036, and by associated companies, branches
and representatives throughout the world.

First published 1985

ISBN 0-443-02564-9

British Library Cataloguing in Publication Data
Manual of haematology.
    1. Blood — diseases
    I. Baughan, Annabelle S.J.
    616.1'5   RC636

Library of Congress Cataloging in Publication Data
Manual of haematology.
    (Manuals series)
    ` 1. Blood — Diseases — Handbooks, manuals, etc.
2. Hematology — Handbooks, manuals, etc.   I. Baughan, Annabelle S.J.   II. Series
[DNLM: 1. Hematology — handbooks. WH 39 M294]
RC636.M35   1985   616.1'5   85-11286

MANUAL OF HAEMATOLOGY

Already published

Paediatric Gastroenterology *J.H. Tripp and D.C.A. Candy*
Renal Disease *C.B. Brown*

Forthcoming volumes in the Manuals series

Clinical Blood Transfusion *M. Brozovic and B. Brozovic*
Gastroenterology *B.T. Cooper and R.E. Barry*
Cardiology *K. Dawkins*
Infection Control *A.M. Emmerson, E.A. Jenner and V.E. Todd*
Infectious Diseases *J.A. Innes*
Rheumatology *J.M.H. Moll*
Chest Medicine *J.E. Stark, J.M. Shneerson, C.D.R. Flower and T. Higenbottam*
Neonatal Intensive Care *A.R. Wilkinson*

PREFACE

This manual is a guide to the practical management of patients with haematological disorders. It is particularly intended to be used by the house officer, senior house officer and registrar grades. The authors, all of whom are practising clinical haematologists, have attempted to express a consensus opinion on the more controversial aspects of clinical management. Nevertheless, practice in different units will vary, and junior staff are urged to liaise with their local laboratory and haematologist over the more difficult clinical decisions.

Appropriate investigations are detailed in each chapter. Although performing all investigations at once may produce quick results, this is at great cost to the diagnostic departments, and subjects the patient to unnecessary tests. Except in the more urgent clinical situations, a more logical approach is to review one batch of test results before ordering another.

We would like thank Mrs M.A. Patterson, Miss Jane Morris and Mrs Margaret Geary for secretarial assistance. We also thank our publishers, Churchill Livingstone, for their patience during the preparation of the manuscript.

Although chapters are included on blood component therapy and acute transfusion reactions there is a more comprehensive coverage of these subjects in our companion volume *Manual of Blood Transfusion*.

1985

A.S.J.B.
A.S.B.H.
K.G.P.
L.S.

PREFACE

CONTENTS

GLOSSARY OF ABBREVIATIONS

AL	Acute leukaemia
ALL	Acute lymphoblastic leukaemia
AML	Acute myeloblastic leukaemia
APTT	Activated partial thromboplastin time
AT III	Anti-thrombin III
BMT	Bone marrow transplantation
cALL	Common acute lymphoblastic leukaemia (antigen)
CGL	Chronic granulocytic leukaemia
CLL	Chronic lymphocytic leukaemia
CMML	Chronic myelo-monocytic leukaemia
DAT	Direct anti-globulin (Coombs) test
DDAVP	DesAmino D-arginine vasopressin
DIC	Disseminated intravascular coagulation
ESR	Erthrocyte sedimentation rate
FFP	Fresh frozen plasma
Hb	Haemoglobin
HD	Hodgkins disease
HLA	Human leukocyte antigen ('tissue type')
HTLV	Human T-cell leukaemia virus
ITP	Idiopathic thrombocytopenic purpura
MAHA	Microangiopathic haemolytic anaemia
MCH	Mean corpuscular haemoglobin
MCHC	Mean corpuscular haemoglobin concentration
MCV	Mean corpuscular volume
MDS	Myelodysplastic syndrome
NAP	Neutrophil alkaline phosphatase
NHL	Non-Hodgkins lymphoma
NSAID	Non-steroidal anti-inflammatory drug
PA	Pernicious anaemia
PLL	ProLymphocytic leukaemia
PPF	Plasma protein fraction
PRV	Polycythaemia rubra vera
PT	Prothrombin time
RAEB	Refractory anaemia with excess of blasts
RBC	Red blood (cell) count
SAA	Severe aplastic anaemia
SCD	Sickle cell disease
sIg	Surface marker immunoglobulin
TT	Thrombin time

Part 1
ANAEMIA

1. A GENERAL APPROACH TO ANAEMIA

DEFINITION OF ANAEMIA

A reduction in haemoglobin level in the blood. *True anaemia* occurs when this is due to a decrease in the circulating red cell mass. *Spurious anaemia* may result from the dilutional effect of an increase in plasma volume in pregnancy, cardiac failure, fluid overload and massive splenomegaly.

CAUSES

1. Blood loss.
2. Increased destruction i.e. haemolysis.
3. Failure of production:
   a. Nutritional deficiencies — iron (p. 9), vitamin B12, folic acid (p. 16), ascorbic acid.
   b. Reduction in erythroid precursors — aplasia (p. 79) bone marrow infiltration (Ch. 5), leukaemia (Chs 18,19) carcinoma, myeloma (Ch. 21), lymphoma (Ch. 22), myelofibrosis (Ch. 5).
   c. Ineffective erythropoiesis: failure of apparently active erythropoiesis to result in adequate numbers of circulating red cells:
      (i) Anaemia of chronic disease.
      (ii) Endocrine failure — thyroid, pituitary.
      (iii) Renal failure.
      (iv) Sideroblastic anaemia.
      (v) Myelodysplastic syndromes.
      (vi) Thalassaemias.

Many conditions cause anaemia by more than one mechanism, e.g. thalassaemia causes both haemolysis and ineffective erythropoiesis; myelofibrosis may cause anaemia by ineffective erythropoiesis, displacement of erythroid cells by reticulin and a dilutional anaemia because of splenic pooling; disseminated cancer may result in blood loss, bone marrow infiltration and anaemia of chronic disease.

3

CLINICAL MANIFESTATIONS

Severity of clinical symptoms depends on:
1. Severity of anaemia.
2. Speed of onset — gradual onset is better tolerated.
3. Age and cardiovascular status of patient — young tolerate anaemia better than elderly.
4. Degree of reduction in O_2 carrying capacity e.g. HbS gives better tissue oxygenation than HbA and the low Hb in sickle cell anaemia therefore is better tolerated.

Symptoms

Fatigue, dyspnoea, faintness, palpitations, dizziness, headache, blackouts, angina, oedema.

Signs

Pallor of mucous membranes and skin creases, tachycardia, heart failure.
   In profound chronic anaemia: retinal haemorrhages and papilloedema, splenomegaly, mild fever.
   Other clinical observations may be suggestive of aetiology.

Points to note in history

1. Previous blood tests — for recent comparison.
2. Duration of symptoms — recent or longstanding.
3. Family history — e.g. congenital haemolytic anaemia, pernicious anaemia.
4. Operations — gastrectomy; small bowel surgery.
5. Drugs — aspirin and NSAIDs causing haemolysis. or aplasia (see Ch. 35).
6. Exposure to toxic chemicals — haemolysis, aplasia.
7. Abdominal symptoms — splenomegaly, GI blood loss, malabsorption, GI neoplasm.
8. Urinary symptoms — renal failure, dark urine in haemolysis.
9. Menstrual and obstetric history — iron deficiency.
10. Blood loss — nose bleeds, GI loss.
11. Dietary history — iron, folate and B12 intake.
12. Oral symptoms — sore tongue, oral ulcers, fissures at angles of mouth.
13. Neurological symptoms — paraesthesiae.
14. Abnormal bruising.
15. Bone pain.

Points to note on examination

1. Racial group — pernicious anaemia, sickle cell disease, thalassaemia.
2. Skin and sclerae — pallor, jaundice, purpura and bruises, telangiectases.
3. Nails — ridging, pitting and koilonychia.
4. Cardiovascular — heart failure, tachycardia, systolic murmurs.
5. Lymph nodes — enlarged.
6. Abdomen — distension, ascites, enlarged liver or spleen, masses.
7. Rectal examination — GI blood loss, melaena stool, masses.

INVESTIGATIONS

Blood count

To include:
1. WBC, RBC, Hb, MCV, MCH, MCHC, platelets.
2. Blood film.
3. Reticulocyte count.

On the basis of the red cell count and indices and examination of red cells on the film, three main types of anaemia may be discerned:

1. Hypochromic, microcytic
   a. RBC count relatively high compared to Hb.
   b. MCV low.
   c. MCH low.
   d. MCHC slightly reduced.
   e. Red cells poorly haemoglobinished on film.
2. Macrocytic
   a. RBC count relatively low compared to Hb.
   b. MCV raised.
   c. MCH raised.
   d. MCHC moderately raised.
   e. Cells large and well haemoglobinised on film.
3. Normochromic, normocytic
   MCV, MCH, MCHC normal.

For further investigation of these three main groups see subsequent chapters. Examination of the red cells on the blood film may reveal other morphological changes which may be of use, e.g. nucleated red cells — suggestive of haemolytic (Ch. 6) or leucoerythroblastic anaemia (Ch. 5) or spherocytes, elliptocytes or red cell fragments (p 243).

Reticulocyte count in anaemia

Raised reticulocyte count suggests:
1. Haemorrhage.
2. Haemolysis.
3. Nutritional deficiency responding to treatment.

Very low reticulocyte count suggests:
1. Hypoplasia or aplasia.
2. Extensive marrow infiltration.

Leucocyte count in anaemia
1. Neutrophil leucocytosis — bleeding or haemolysis, infections.
2. Neutrophil left shift — seen in leuco-erythroblastic anaemias (with nucleated red cells) (Ch.5).
3. Primitive WBC e.g. blasts — leukaemias, myeloproliferative disorders, leuco-erythroblastic anaemia.
4. Leucopenia — bone marrow aplasia or infiltration, megaloblastic anaemia, immune disorders, e.g. Felty's syndrome, SLE, hypersplenism.
5. Hypersegmented neutrophils — megaloblastic anaemias.

Platelet count in anaemia

Thrombocytosis suggests:
1. Bleeding
2. Haemolysis.
3. Myeloproliferative disorders.
4. Iron deficiency with or without bleeding.

Thrombocytopenia suggests:
1. Bone marrow aplasia or infiltration.
2. Megaloblastic anaemia.

Other investigations

1. Serum iron and total iron binding capacity } iron
2. Serum ferritin } status.
3. Serum vitamin B12 and folate if macrocytosis present.
4. Renal function (urea, creatinine, electrolytes).
5. Liver function test (bilirubin, hepatic enzymes, alkaline phosphatase, urinary urobilinogen).
6. Thyroid function if hypothyroidism suspected.
7. A bone marrow is indicated ($\pm$trephine biopsy)
   a. If one of the following is suspected:
      Megaloblastic change.
      Leukaemias.
      Bone marrow infiltration.
      Myeloma.
      Myelodysplastic or myeloproliferative syndromes.
      Sideroblastic anaemia.
      Aplasia or hypoplasia.

b. As an absolute index of iron status where there is doubt about diagnosis.

c. In other anaemias of uncertain aetiology.

A bone marrow is not indicated in simple iron deficiency and most cases of anaemia secondary to chronic disease. For futher investigations see subsequent chapters.

TREATMENT

1. Elucidate the cause and treat appropriately.
2. If anaemia is secondary to underlying systemic disease, treatment of the disease, if possible, will improve the anaemia. Inappropriate use of haematinics is useless. The anaemia per se may not be symptomatic or require treatment.
3. Symptomatic transfusion may be required.
   a. In acute blood loss transfuse as appropriate to the patient's vital signs; Hb level may not provide a useful indication of amount of blood loss.
   b. In chronic anaemia do not transfuse if the haemoglobin is stable and not giving rise to symptoms. Where anaemia is progressive, transfuse with packed cells to Hb level desired. In an adult one unit of blood will raise Hb by approximately 1 g/dl. Do not initiate regular transfusions unless there is a clear indication that the patient will benefit. See Chapter 29 on blood transfusion for details.
4. Heart failure should be treated appropriately with diuretics and rest.

REFERENCE

Cawley J C, McNicol G P 1979 The investigation of the anaemic patient. British Journal of Hospital Medicine Aug:158–167

2. HYPOCHROMIC MICROCYTIC ANAEMIA

DEFINITION

A low haemoglobin with hypochromic microcytic red cells on the blood film, a low MCV and a low MCH.

CAUSES

1. Iron deficiency.
2. Hereditary haemoglobin disorders.
3. Anaemia secondary to chronic disorders or renal failure.
4. Sideroblastic anaemia.

INITIAL INVESTIGATIONS

1. Hb, MCV, MCH, red cell count and morphology.
2. Platelet count, reticulocyte count and ESR.
3. Serum for iron and TIBC measurement.

INVESTIGATIONS SOMETIMES REQUIRED

1. Haemoglobin electrophoresis with HbA_2 level.
2. Marrow aspiration to assess red cell morphology and iron stores and to exclude sideroblastic anaemia.
3. Supravital stain of blood film to exclude $\propto$-thalassaemia. Globin chain synthesis if available.
4. Appropriate tests dictated by clinical findings to exclude renal failure, collagen diseases, etc.
5. Iron deficiency is not a diagnosis in itself and appropriate investigations to establish its cause should be undertaken.

INTERPRETATION OF RESULTS

See Table 2.1.

IRON DEFICIENCY

By far the most common cause of anaemia in the world.

Stages of progressive iron deficiency
Distinct tissue iron deficiency can be present despite a normal haemoglobin and red cell indices.

1. Normal Hb, serum iron and TIBC. Low ferritin. Absent marrow stainable iron.
2. Reduced serum iron and raised TIBC.
3. Low MCV and/or MCH on automated blood counter.
4. Hypochromic microcytes in the blood film.
5. Anaemia.
6. Reduced MCHC.
7. Epithelial changes.

Increasing iron deficiency.

Tissue effects of iron deficiency
1. Adults: Dry, fine, brittle, prematurely greyed hair. Skin pigmentation. Brittle, ridged nails. Koilonychia. Smooth sore tongue. Angular stomatitis. Occasional splenomegaly. Retinal oedema with haemorrhages, occasionally papilloedema. Postcricoid web with dysphagia. Gastritis with gastric atrophy and achlorhydria.
2. Children: Anorexia. Pica. Failure to thrive. Splenomegaly in 10%. Repeated respiratory infections. Epithelial changes rare.

Important clinical features in establishing the cause of iron deficiency
1. Genito-urinary: Frequency and duration of periods and amount of menstrual blood loss. Dark or bloodstained urine, renal colic. Primary infertility (coeliac disease). Number of pregnancies.
2. Gastrointestinal: Abdominal pain (peptic ulceration, gastric carcinoma, hiatus hernia). Vomiting (Mallory-Weiss). Fatty stools (malabsorption). Altered bowel habit (diverticulitis, colon carcinoma). Jaundice (varices, coagulopathy).
3. Overt blood loss from any site.
4. Past medical history: previous iron deficiency, gastrectomy, duodenal bypass, regular blood donor, prosthetic heart valve, chronic liver disease.

Table 2.1

	Iron deficiency	Thalassaemia trait	Anaemia of chronic disease	Sideroblastic anaemia
MCV, MCH	Reduced in proportion to severity of anaemia	Reduced. Very low for degree of anaemia	Only slight reduction	Low, normal or raised
Red cell count	Reduced	Increased	Reduced	Reduced
Serum iron	Reduced	Normal/increased	Reduced	Increased
TIBC	Increased	Normal	Reduced	Reduced
ESR	Normal/increased	Normal	Increased	Normal
Reticulocyte count	Any	Increased/normal	Reduced	Normal/reduced
Marrow macrophage iron stores	Absent	Increased/normal	Increased	Increased
Marrow erythroblast iron	Absent	Increased/normal	Reduced	Increased — ring forms
Haemoglobin A2	Falsely low	Increased (β) Reduced ($\propto$)	Normal	Normal

5. Drugs: Anti-inflammatory drugs, corticosteroids, anti-coagulants, aspirin (ask about proprietary compounds containing salicylates).
6. Diet: Foods rich in iron — red meat, soyabean protein, fish, egg yolk, green vegetables, fruit. Factors diminishing iron absorption — cereals, eggs, chapatis, tea, long-term tetracycline treatment.
7. Alcohol intake: Poor diet, gastritis, coagulopathy.
8. Travel abroad: Hookworm (endemic in Central and South America, Africa, Oceania), Schistosoma haematobium, Trichuris trichiura.
9. Family history: Coagulation disorders, hereditary haemorrhagic telangiectasia, Peutz-Jeghers.
10. Skin: Bruising, petechiae, stigmata of chronic liver disease, Peutz-Jegher spots.

Blood and marrow changes

1. Red cells: small and pale, pencil cells, target cells, anisocytosis and poikilocytosis.
2. Increased platelet count and mild neutropenia.
3. Marrow shows increased numbers of red cell precursors, poor haemoglobinization and no stainable iron.

Useful tests to establish cause of bleeding

1. Faeces:
   a. Occult bloods (can be unreliable and do not exclude intermittent bleeding).
   b. Ova and parasites.
2. Blood tests:
   a. Liver function tests (coagulopathy, variceal bleeding).
   b. Thyroid function tests (menorrhagia common in myxoedema).
   c. Eosinophil count (intestinal parasites).
   d. Blood film for hyposplenic features (coeliac disease).
   e. Coagulation screen.
3. Urine:
   a. Microscopy (microscopic haematuria).
   b. Haemosiderin (chronic intravascular haemolysis).
4. X-rays:
   a. Barium swallow (hiatus hernia, varices, carcinoma, post-cricoid web).
   b. Barium meal (ulcer, carcinoma, benign tumour).
   c. Barium follow-through (Meckel's diverticulum, polyps).
   d. IVP if haematuria present.
   e. Selective angiography.

5. As indicated:
   a. Endoscopy.
   b. Jejunal biopsy.
   c. Occasionally, exploratory laparotomy is required in persistent undiagnosed gastrointestinal blood loss.

TREATMENT

N.B. Treat the underlying cause

Oral iron

1. The route of choice.
2. Avoid slow-release preparations (poorly absorbed).
3. Avoid mixed vitamin compounds (treat the specific deficiency only).
4. Choose the cheapest preparation.
5. Give as a divided dose to minimise the side effects (t.d.s. is probably best).
6. Initially, prescribe oral iron to be taken before meals. If this causes gastric intolerance, change to 'after meals' (but this will reduce the absorption).
7. There is no proven reduction in the incidence of side-effects with any one preparation, although one form may be better tolerated than another by an individual patient.
8. Side-effects: Black motions, (will not affect results of occult blood testing), nausea, epigastric pain, diarrhoea or constipation.
9. Give 150–200 mg elemental iron daily e.g. ferrous sulphate B.P. (200 mg = 60 mg elemental iron, 3–4 tablets daily) or ferrous gluconate BP (300 mg = 36 mg elemental iron, 5–6 tablets daily) or ferrous fumarate BP (200 mg = 65 mg elemental iron, 2–3 tablets daily) (particularly useful for patients with small children as the tablets are not sugar coated and therefore less likely to be mistaken for sweets).
10. Optimal response: rise in haemoglobin of one g/dl per week.
11. Continue treatment for three months after the haemoglobin has returned to normal to replenish the body iron stores.
12. Justifications for prophylactic oral iron: partial or total gastrectomy, low birth-weight infants, pregnancy, female blood donors.
13. Failure of response to oral iron: wrong diagnosis (suspect thalassaemia trait), patient not taking the tablets, persisting blood loss, intestinal malabsorption, chronic disease states which will impair the marrow response to iron.

Parenteral iron

1. Justifications: genuine intolerance of oral iron, failure of oral iron in malabsorptive states, ileostomy (when oral iron may cause offensive diarrhoea), occasionally when a patient is unreliable about taking tablets.
2. The haemoglobin response is *no faster* with parenteral iron compared to oral iron that is reliably taken and normally absorbed.
3. Approximate total dose needed = (15.0 − Hb level) × 250 mg.

Intramuscular iron

1. Give as deep i.m. injection in the upper outer quadrant of the buttock by Z track technique.
2. Recommended preparation: iron sorbitol ('Jectofer').
3. Contains 50 mg iron/ml. First dose 1 ml, followed by daily 1 or 2 ml according to tolerance.
4. Side-effects: skin staining if the dose leaks along the needle track, occasional nausea and vomiting, fever, swelling of local lymph nodes, joint pains, metallic taste in the mouth.

Intravenous iron

1. To be avoided unless absolutely necessary e.g. if emaciation or coagulation defect preclude intramuscular injection or if patient is unlikely to attend for a course of i.m. injections.
2. Contra-indicated in any patient with a history of allergy e.g. hay fever, asthma, previous drug reactions.
3. Given as iron dextran ('Imferon'). 'Jectofer' must not be given intravenously.
4. Administration: Consult the chart that comes with the pack for the dose required. Dilute in 250–500 ml of 5% dextrose or normal saline and give as an infusion over 6–8 hours. The drip must be started very slowly and the doctor should remain with the patient for the first ten minutes. Thereafter, the patient must be under close nursing supervision. Severe anaphylactic reactions may occur with i.v. iron — always have adrenaline and Pirition at hand (skin testing is unfortunately of no value in predicting adverse reactions).
5. Other side-effects: phlebitis at the site of the injection, nausea, vomiting, headache, pyrexia.

HEREDITARY HAEMOGLOBIN DISORDERS CAUSING HYPOCHROMIC MICROCYTIC ANAEMIA

ß-thalassaemia trait

1. Asymptomatic. Usually discovered on routine blood tests.
2. Very common, especially in patients from Mediterranean countries, South-East Asia, Middle East, Far East and India but by no means rare in North Europeans.
3. Blood findings
   a. Normal or slightly low haemoglobin.
   b. Marked reduction in MCV (often less than 65 fl).
   c. Marked reduction in MCH (often less than 24 pgm).
   d. Raised or high-normal red cell count.
   e. Film shows hypochromic microcytes and/or occasional target cells and/or basophilic stippling.
   f. Raised HbA_2 level to more than 3.5%.
4. Patient with ß-thalassaemia trait can be coincidentally iron deficient. It is useful to measure the serum iron and TIBC in each suspected case, particularly as iron deficiency will give a falsely low HbA_2 result.
5. Advise each newly diagnosed patient:
   a. That it will not cause them any symptoms.
   b. That their spouse should be tested for thalassaemia trait too. If they both have it, their offspring each have a one-in-four liklihood of having ß-thalassaemia major — a devastating disease. Offer such couples genetic counselling and ante-natal diagnosis early in pregnancy (requires referral to a specialist centre).
   c. That they should tell any doctor they see that they have ß-thalassaemia trait. This should prevent them being given unnecessary iron treatment because of the findings of a low MCV and MCH. Such patients not uncommonly present with iatrogenic iron overload.
6. No treatment is necessary except that folic acid tablets should be given at times of acute marrow stress e.g. bleeding, pregnancy.

∝-thalassaemia trait

1. The genetics are more complicated than in ß-thalassaemia so that the term 'trait' is usually applied to mild clinical phenotypes.
2. Common in the Far East (particularly Thailand) but also seen in people of Mediterranean, Asian and African origin.
3. Asymptomatic

4. Blood findings:
   a. Haemoglobin normal or slightly reduced.
   b. Low MCV and MCH.
   c. Raised red cell count.
   d. Normal HbA_2 and occasionally raised HbF.
   e. Supravital staining of the blood film may show 'golf-ball' red cells containing HbH inclusions. Such cells may be very scanty (1 in 1000–3000).
5. The diagnosis can usually be proven with globin chain synthesis analysis but this is not commonly available. $\propto$-thalassaemia trait can be assumed to be present in a patient with hypochromic microcytic red cells, normal HbA_2, normal iron studies and identical findings in a first-degree relative.
6. Management: As for ß-thalassaemia trait.

SIDEROBLASTIC ANAEMIA

1. To be suspected in a patient with a hypochromic microcytic anaemia but a high serum iron and ferritin and low TIBC (it more usually causes a macrocytic or dimorphic anaemia).
2. Can be diagnosed only by bone marrow aspiration to demonstrate the presence of abnormal ringed sideroblasts.
3. Causes: Hereditary sex-linked, idiopathic acquired, drugs, alcohol, rarely with collagen disorders.
4. Treatment: Remove cause if known. Idiopathic cases may respond to oral folic acid and pyridoxine, but they usually require a chronic blood transfusion regime.

ANAEMIA OF CHRONIC DISORDERS

This is usually normochromic and normocytic, but if severe and prolonged can become mildly hypochromic microcytic. Generally the haemoglobin does not fall below 8 g/dl. The findings include reduced serum iron, reduced TIBC, increased marrow reticulo-endothelial iron but reduced erythroblast iron, and a high ESR. The anaemia will respond to successful treatment of the underlying condition and will not respond to iron treatment.

REFERENCE

Jacobs A (ed) 1982 Disorders of iron metabolism. Clinics in Haematology 11(2):

3. MACROCYTOSIS AND MACROCYTIC ANAEMIA

DEFINITION

A raised MCV usually > 100fl (depending on the blood counter used), associated with a significant number of large red cells on the blood film. Macrocytosis may commonly be present without anaemia.

CAUSES

Macrocytosis associated with a megaloblastic marrow

Blood film usually shows oval macrocytes, and poikilocytosis can be prominent. Hypersegmented (> 5 lobes) polymorphs are usually seen, and there can often be modest decreases in both leucocyte and platelet counts. Sometimes the blood appearances are sufficiently characteristic to make a marrow unnecessary in initial diagnostic work up.

Vitamin B12 deficiency

1. *Nutritional*
   Particularly strict vegans (e.g. Hindus).
2. *Gastric malabsorption*
   Intrinsic factor, secreted by the gastric mucosa, is necessary for the absorption of B12 in the terminal ileum. Lack of intrinsic factor may cause B12 deficiency in pernicious anamia (PA) — the commonest cause of B12 deficiency in western countries — and after partial or total gastrectomy.
3. *Intestinal malabsorption*
   Ileal resection or Crohn's disease of the terminal ileum may remove absorptive capacity.
   Bacterial colonisation of the small intestine by micro-organisms that consume B12 may competitively impair absorption e.g. bacteria in small intestinal diverticulae or stagnant loop.
4. *Drugs*
   Usually lead to minor malabsorption only e.g. PAS, colchicine, neomycin, phenformin.

Folic acid deficiency
1. Nutritional
   a. Poverty, especially in the elderly.
   b. Alcoholics.
2. Malabsorption
   a. Gluten sensitive enteropathy.
   b. Tropical sprue.
3. Increased requirements
   a. Physiological: Pregnancy, infants.
   b. Pathological: Malignancies, chronic haemolytic anaemia (especially thalassaemia and sickle cell disease), myelofibrosis, chronic inflammatory disease (e.g. rheumatoid arthritis).
4. Drugs
   a. Cholestyramine (due to decreased absorption)
   b. Anticonvulsants (mechanism uncertain)
   c. Alcohol (especially if associated with liver disease).
5. Increased loss
   a. Removal in haemodialysis fluid.
6. Liver disease.

Causes of megaloblastic change not associated with B12 or folate deficiency
1. Erythroleukaemia (megaloblastic change associated with increased blasts).
2. Sideroblastic anaemia (marrow may be megaloblastic or normoblastic but iron stain reveals ring sideroblasts).
3. Alcohol (direct toxic effect on marrow erythroid cells).
4. Drugs which interfere with nucleic acid metabolism e.g. methotrexate, pyrimethamine, trimethoprin, cytosine arabinoside.

Macrocytosis associated with a normoblastic marrow

Macrocytes tend to be round, not oval. They may be polychromatic (p. 245) indicating a reticulocytosis.

There is no neutrophil nuclear hypersegmentation.

Causes

1. Reticulocytosis (young red cells are large red cells) associated with haemolysis or bleeding.
2. Aplastic anaemia and pure red cell aplasia.
3. Liver disease. Target cells (p. 244) are commonly seen on the film.
4. Alcohol.
5. Myxoedema, but check not due to associated PA.
6. Sideroblastic anaemia (p. 15).
7. Myeloid leukaemias and myelo-dysplastic syndromes.
8. Chronic respiratory failure.

CLINICAL ASSESSMENT

1. Fair hair (or premature greying) and blue eyes are typically found in PA.
2. Sore tongue is not specific but suggests B12 or folate deficiency.
3. Peripheral parasthesiae and difficulty in walking suggest the peripheral neuropathy of B12 deficiency.
4. PA often associated with vitiligo and auto-immune thyroid and adrenal disease.
5. Take a simple dietary history, including alcohol intake.
6. Ask about a past history of gastro-intestinal disease or operations, and ask about steatorrhoea.
7. Ascertain whether there is a history of haemolytic disease, myelofibrosis or chronic disease.
8. Take a drug history.
9. Psychiatric disturbances may occur in B12 and folate deficiency.
10. Coeliac disease may be suggested by a history of skin rash (dermatitis herpetiformis), primary infertility, or small stature compared with siblings.

LABORATORY ASSESSMENT

Initial investigations
Hb, MCV, white cell and platelet counts with blood film. If these suggest megaloblastic anaemia or there is clinical suspicion of B12 or folate deficiency it may be necessary to do a bone marrow aspirate — consult with the haematologist. Marrow should always be stained for iron to assess iron stores and look for ring sideroblasts.

Measurement of serum B12 and folate levels
This may be performed by microbiological assay or radioassay. The former may give falsely low results if the patient is on antibiotics or cytotoxics.

With either assay increased B12 levels can be found in:
1. *Leucocytosis.*
   May be associated with myeloproliferative disorders particularly chronic granulocytic leukaemia. The B12 level is usually normal in benign granulocytosis.
2. *Active liver disease.*

In B12 deficiency there is a decreased serum B12 and often a decreased red cell folate and increased serum folate.

In folate deficiency serum and red cell folate are decreased with a normal or slightly reduced B12.

Red cell folate levels give a better guide to tissue folate stores than serum folate.

Investigations to establish the cause of B12 deficiency

1. Schilling test to investigate B12 absorption. This should be done after effective parenteral therapy of B12 deficiency.

   Part I Give 1000 μg of non-radioactive B12 i.m. and 1 μg of radioactive B12 by mouth. Collect the urine over a 24 hour period. Normally > 10% of the ingested radioactivity appears in the urine. If abnormal:

   Part II Repeat as for Part I but give oral intrinsic factor as well as radioactive B12.

   With PA there is an increase in the percentage of radioactivity excreted, compared to Part I, but not with intestinal malabsorption.

   These tests can be carried out within 48 hours of one another, and have been combined commercially as the 'Dicopac' test.

2. Serum antibodies to gastric parietal cells (not very specific to PA), and intrinsic factor (more specific to PA, but found less commonly).

   Other auto-antibodies may be found in PA as there is an association with autoimmune thyroid and adrenal disease.

3. Barium meal and follow through. The follow through may demonstrate small intestinal lesions such as terminal ileal disease or diverticuli. Gastric atrophy is common in PA and there is a higher incidence of gastric carcinoma.

Investigations to establish the cause of folate deficiency

1. Investigation of intestinal absorption e.g. barium follow through, xylose tolerance test (5 hour urine collection after 5g of oral xylose — consult biochemistry laboratory), jejunal biopsy (necessary for the diagnosis of coeliac disease).

2. Other tests as appropriate, looking for evidence of an underlying disease (see above).

3. Serum IgA may be decreased in coeliac disease.

Investigation of macrocytosis with a normoblastic marrow

1. The marrow may reveal leukaemia, sideroblastic anaemia (iron stain necessary), hypoplasia or pure red cell aplasia. In aplastic anaemia a trephine biopsy is necessary to establish hypoplasia.

2. Reticulocyte count.

3. Liver function tests.

4. Thyroid function tests.

A pragmatic approach to macrocytic anaemia

An appropriate initial assessment of the patient with macrocytic anaemia includes:

1. B12 and folate levels.
2. Reticulocyte count.
3. Liver function tests.
4. Thyroid function test.

Further investigations are then dictated by the B12 and folate levels.

TREATMENT

B12 deficiency

Vitamin B12 (hydroxycobalamin) is relatively inexpensive and non-toxic — overdosage does no harm. With PA or malabsorption give 1000 μg hydroxycobalamin weekly for six weeks, then every three months for life.

Following initial treatment there is a reticulocyte response between days five and seven.

After correction of deficiency by parenteral therapy vegans can be given an oral daily maintenance dose of 50 μg B12.

Folate deficiency

Folic acid 5 mg daily by mouth for four months or longer, depending on cause. With severe malabsorption may need 15 mg daily initially.

Long term folic acid is usually only required with chronic haemolytic anaemias and myelofibrosis.

Prophylactic folic acid should be administered to pregnant women, premature babies and patients on regular haemodialysis.

Severe megaloblastic anaemia

Perform a bone marrow and collect blood for B12 and folate estimations. Then give both B12 and folic acid (folic acid alone given to a B12 deficient patient can precipitate neurological damage). Blood transfusion is dangerous in patients with severe megaloblastic anaemia and should be reserved for those exceptional patients with anoxic symptoms e.g. angina. Use 1–2 units of packed cells given slowly with diuretic cover. The plasma potassium level should be monitored as it tends to drop with effective B12 therapy in severe megaloblastic anaemia.

REFERENCES

Parry T E 1980 The diagnosis of megaloblastic anaemia. Clinical and Laboratory Haematology 2: 89–109
Sullivan L W 1970 Differential diagnosis and management of the patient with megaloblastic anaemia. American Journal of Medicine 48: 609–615

4. NORMOCHROMIC NORMOCYTIC ANAEMIA

DEFINITION

A low haemoglobin in the presence of a normal MCV, MCH and MCHC.

Anaemia of chronic disease

When a normocytic, normochromic anaemia is due to underlying inflammation, neoplasia or longstanding infection it is also known as 'anaemia of chronic disease', 'secondary anaemia' or 'symptomatic anaemia'. The majority of these patients will have obvious evidence of the underlying disease.

CAUSES

1. Anaemia with inadequate marrow response
   a. Disturbed iron utilization
      (i)   Anaemia of chronic disorders
      (ii) Sideroblastic anaemia (occasionally)
   b. Intrinsic bone marrow disease or infiltration
      (i)   Hypoplastic anaemia
      (ii) Metastatic carcinoma
      (iii) Leukaemia, lymphoma, myeloma
   c. Decreased erythropoietin drive
      (i)   Chronic renal failure
      (ii) Various endocrine disorders e.g. myxoedema, Addison's.
2. Anaemia with appropriate marrow response
   a. Acute haemorrhage
   b. Haemolysis.

IMPORTANT POINTS TO NOTE IN HISTORY AND EXAMINATION

The patient with anaemia secondary to chronic disease will virtually always be symptomatic of the underlying disease.

Malignant tumours have not been included in this list as they may give rise to any symptom or sign.

1. General
   a. Overt bleeding (acute haemorrhage, aplasia, leukaemia)
   b. Purpura (liver disease, leukaemia, renal failure)
   c. Weight loss (TB, SBE, Addisons disease)
   d. Fever (infection, collagen disorder, leukaemia)
   e. Jaundice (haemolysis, liver disease)
   f. Rash (collagen disorders, lymphoma)
   g. Lymphadenopathy (leukaemia, lymphoma)
   h. Goitre (myxoedema)
   i. Pruritus (renal failure, lymphoma)
   j. Finger clubbing (SBE, lung abscess, cirrhosis).
2. Abdomen
   a. Diarrhoea (Addisons, infective)
   b. Constipation (myxoedema)
   c. Nausea and vomiting (chronic renal failure, Addison's)
   d. Pain (pelvic inflammatory disease, recurrent UTIs)
   e. Hepatosplenomegaly (leukaemia, lymphoma, collagen disorders).
3. Cardiorespiratory system
   a. Murmurs (SBE)
   b. Tachycardia (some infections, Addisons)
   c. Pericarditis (SLE, TB, Rheumatoid disease)
   d. Cough, dyspnoea (pulmonary TB, collagen disorders, lung abscess).
4. Genitourinary system
   a. Polyuria, nocturia (chronic renal failure)
   b. Dysuria (recurrent urinary tract infections)
   c. Vaginal discharge (pelvic inflammatory disease).
5. Central nervous system
   a. Focal signs (leukaemia, lymphoma).
6. Musculo-skeletal system
   a. Bone pain (myeloma, leukaemia, osteomyelitis)
   b. Joint pain (collagen disorders).
7. Drug history, particularly those that can cause marrow hypoplasia, haemolysis, bleeding diathesis, renal failure (Ch. 35).

INVESTIGATIONS

1. Full blood count including platelet count, white cell count and differential, blood film morphology.
2. Reticulocyte count.
3. ESR.
4. Serum iron and TIBC.
5. Plasma urea, creatinine and electrolytes.
6. Liver function tests.
7. Chest X-ray.
8. Other investigations as clinically indicated e.g. MSU, blood cultures, auto-antibodies, Mantoux test, ferritin, thyroid function.
9. Bone marrow aspirate and trephine biopsy, if underlying cause not obvious.

INTERPRETATION OF INVESTIGATIONS

1. Haemoglobin
   In anaemia of chronic disease the haemoglobin is not usually less than 8g/dl.
2. White cell count
   a. Neutrophilia; blood loss, infection, disseminated malignancy
   b. Abnormal white cells: leukaemia, lymphoma
   c. Neutropenia: aplastic anaemia, SLE, overwhelming sepsis, some leukaemias.
3. ESR
   a. Usually normal in haemorrhage, endocrinopathies
   b. Normal or increased in liver disease, renal failure
   c. Usually increased in myeloma, collagen disorders, metastatic carcinoma, haematological malignancy, various infections particularly TB.
4. Reticulocyte count
   a. Normal or reduced: infection, aplasia, renal failure, endocrinopathies
   b. Normal or moderately increased: malignancy, marrow infiltration, liver disease
   c. Increased to 5–15%: blood loss, haemolysis
   d. Increased to > 15%: haemolysis.
5. Serum iron and TIBC
   a. ↓ iron ↑ TIBC: iron deficiency
   b. ↓ iron ↓ TIBC: anaemia of chronic disorders
   c. ↑ iron ↓ TIBC: chronic haemolysis
   d. Both normal: acute haemorrhage, some endocrinopathies.

MANAGEMENT OF NORMOCHROMIC NORMOCYTIC ANAEMIA

1. Correct the underlying cause.
2. Blood transfusion
   a. Indicated:
      (i) to replace blood loss
      (ii) aplastic anaemia, leukaemia or other marrow infiltration
   b. Usually not indicated in renal failure (p. 229) or anaemia of chronic disease as the haemoglobin commonly falls rapidly to the pre-transfusion level.
3. Treatment with iron is contraindicated except in rare cases where iron deficiency (no stainable iron in the bone marrow) is proven. Iron treatment, oral or parenteral, in anaemia of chronic disease will only worsen the reticuloendothelial iron overload and will not improve the haemoglobin.
4. Search carefully for other mechanisms contributing to the anaemia e.g. blood loss in rheumatoid arthritis, folic acid deficiency in liver disease.

REFERENCE

Cartwright G E, Lee G R 1971 The anaemia of chronic disorders. British Journal of Haematology 21: 147–152

5. LEUCOERYTHROBLASTIC ANAEMIA

DEFINITION

The presence in the peripheral blood of nucleated RBC's and immature myeloid cells (metamyelocytes, myelocytes, promyelocytes or even occasionally myeloblasts).

There is a variable degree of anaemia and anisopoikilocytosis. If due to myelofibrosis tear-drop poikilocytes are frequently seen.

CAUSES

1. *Acute marrow stress*
   Seen as part of a marrow response to:
   a. Acute, severe bleeding
   b. Severe haemolysis
   c. Severe infection especially in babies (a leucoerythroblastic picture without anaemia can be seen in healthy neonates)
   The leucoerythroblastic appearances in these patients is usually a transient phenomenon.
2. *Marrow infiltration*
   Most commonly seen with:
   a. Metastatic cancer (especially lung, breast, prostate, kidney, thyroid)
   b. Myelofibrosis (see below)
   c. Myeloma
   d. Lymphoma
   e. Tuberculosis   } Less common.
   f. Lipid storage diseases

The degree of associated anaemia is not quantitatively related to the extent of clinically detectable infiltration. Although conveniently thought of as a 'crowding-out' phenomenon the exact pathogenesis is uncertain. The anaemia is normochromic, normocytic, and is accompanied by variable thrombocytopenia.

CLINICAL ASSESSMENT

1. Bone pain or tenderness to palpation suggests metastases or myeloma.
2. Massive splenomegaly suggests myelofibrosis.
3. Lymphadenopathy and hepato-splenomegaly might indicate a lymphoma, while hepato-splenomegaly alone a storage disease.
4. Mild jaundice with dark urine may suggest haemolysis.
5. Examine breasts, thyroid and do a rectal examination to look for a possible primary carcinoma.
6. Does the patient smoke (bronchogenic carcinoma)?
7. Is there a source of acute bleeding e.g. GIT?

LABORATORY ASSESSMENT

The cause may be obvious from the patient's previous history: if not the following investigations should be carried out:

1. Blood count and film: besides a leucoerythroblastic picture, this may reveal clues as to its cause e.g. tear-drop poikilocytosis in myelofibrosis, rouleaux and occasional plasma cells in myeloma, abnormal lymphoid cells in lymphoma.
2. Bone marrow aspirate and biopsy. A biopsy is mandatory in looking for malignant infiltration and for assessing marrow fibrosis. The marrow can be cultured for TB if this is suspected.
3. Chest X-ray. May reveal primary or metastatic tumour, enlarged hilar lymph nodes or TB.
4. Skeletal survey may demonstrate metastases or myeloma. A bone scan may be helpful in confirming metastases.
5. Serum immunoglobulins, protein electrophoresis and EMU for Bence-Jones protein if myeloma is suspected.

MANAGEMENT

Depends on the underlying disease and its sensitivity to available therapy and the appropriateness of such treatment. Blood transfusion may be required.

MYELOFIBROSIS (Agnogenic myeloid metaplasia)

Myelofibrosis is one of the myeloproliferative disorders that also include polycythaemia rubra vera (p. 60) essential thrombocythaemia (p. 51) and chronic granulocytic leukaemia (p. 111). These disorders are characterised by:
1. A generalised proliferation of bone marrow.
2. Variable marrow fibrosis and extramedullary haemopoiesis in liver and spleen.
3. Morphologically abnormal megakaryocytes.

Polycythaemia shows mainly marrow erythroid hyperplasia with minimal extramedullary erythropoiesis while myelofibrosis has marked extramedullary erythropoiesis with prominent hepato-splenomegaly and marrow fibrosis. In essential thrombocythaemia the megakaryocyte proliferation is particularly prominent. About 25% of patients have syndromes that are transitional between polycythaemia and myelofibrosis.

Clinical features

1. Presents in middle to old age.
2. Insidious onset of symptoms of anaemia which may be due to:
   a. Ineffective erythropoiesis
   b. Splenomegaly causing red cell pooling, decreased red cell survival and dilutional anaemia from increased plasma volume
   c. Folate deficiency due to hyperproliferative marrow.
3. Massive splenomegaly, which may be the presenting symptom.
4. Bleeding manifestations.

Laboratory features

1. Leucoerythroblastic anaemia (see above) with tear-drop poikilocytosis.
2. White cell and platelet counts may be normal, decreased or raised.
3. Bone marrow aspirate is often a 'dry-tap' and a biopsy is required to demonstrate the increased fibrosis.
4. Increased level of serum uric acid (gout is not uncommon) and bilirubin (due to ineffective erythropoiesis).
5. Decreased serum folate.
6. Prolonged bleeding time and impaired platelet function.
7. Isotopic studies (see below).

Management

1. Folic acid 5 mg daily may help maintain haemoglobin.
2. Allopurinol 300 mg p.o. daily if there is high uric acid or cytotoxic treatment is employed.
3. Blood transfusion as required.
4. Low dose single agent cytotoxics (e.g. busulphan) to decrease spleen size or to reduce bone pain or systemic symptoms. Because of impaired marrow reserve patients with myelofibrosis are particularly sensitive to cytotoxic agents and these must be employed with caution.
5. Consider splenectomy or splenic irradiation. Isotope studies measuring plasma volume and sites of red cell production and destruction can be helpful in assessing the potential value of splenectomy. Splenectomy is best undertaken early rather than later in the disease.

   The operation is particularly hazardous because of:
   a. Bleeding tendency (impaired platelet function/ thrombocytopenia).
   b. Adhesions due to small areas of splenic infarction.
   c. Commonly elderly patients.

Course

Usually slowly progressive with increasing anaemia and transfusion requirements. Increasing splenomegaly, weight loss, fever and cachexia occur in the later states. Up to 25% can transform to an acute myeloid leukaemia.

REFERENCES

Burkett L L, Cox M L, Fields M L 1965 Leucoerythroblastosis in the adult. American Journal of Clinical Pathology 44: 494–498
Rojer R A, Mulder N H, Niewig H O 'Classic' and 'acute' myelofibrosis — a retrospective study. Acta Haematologica 60: 108–116

6. HAEMOLYTIC DISORDERS

DEFINITION

Haemolytic disorders are characterised by accelerated red cell destruction usually with a compensatory increase in red cell production. If the rate of destruction exceeds the capacity of the bone marrow to increase production then anaemia results, and increased haemoglobin catabolism leads to jaundice.

CLASSIFICATION

1. Inherited:
   a. Red cell membrane defects e.g. hereditary spherocytosis
   b. Red cell enzyme deficiencies causing membrane instability:
      (i) Asssociated with decreased reducing potential e.g. G6PD deficiency
      (ii) Associated with decreased energy (ATP) production e.g. pyruvate kinase (PK) deficiency
   c. Defects in globin synthesis or structure e.g. thalassaemia, sickle cell disease.
2. Acquired:
   a. Immune:
      (i) Haemolytic disease of the newborn (HDN)
      (ii) Drug associated e.g. methyldopa, penicillin (p. 233)
      (iii) Incompatible blood transfusion (p. 212)
      (iv) Autoimmune
   b. Non-immune:
      (i) Red cell membrane defect — paroxysmal nocturnal haemoglobinuria (PNH)
      (ii) Mechanical disruption: Artifical heart valves, or tight stenosis of a natural heart valve with turbulent blood flow: March haemoglobinuria (Trauma to the red cells in the soles of the feet)

Microangiopathic haemolytic anaemia (MAHA) — caused by intravascular fibrin formation resulting in red cell fragmentation; seen in DIC (p. 175) thrombotic thrombocytopenic purpura, haemolytic uraemic syndrome, malignant hypertension and vasculitis.

(iii) Infections e.g. malaria.

POINTS TO NOTE ON HISTORY AND EXAMINATION

1. Speed of onset of symptoms, history of previous episodes.
2. Presence of jaundice or splenomegaly.
3. Family history of anaemia/jaundice.
4. Stunting of growth, skull bossing, prognathism (children with thalassaemia major and other severe congenital anaemias).
5. Association with infections, drug or food ingestion (G6PD deficiency).
6. Association with cold weather (cold acting antibodies).
7. History of, or presence of, leg ulcers (seen with haemoglobinopathies and hereditary spherocytosis).
8. History of gall-stones/cholecystitis (increased bilirubin excretion).
9. Previous transfusion history.

INVESTIGATIONS

1. Indicating increased red cell destruction:
   a. Increased plasma unconjugated bilirubin
   b. Increased urinary urobilinogen, but absent bilirubin
   c. Haemoglobinuria
   d. Haemosiderinuria } particularly with intra-vascular haemolysis
   e. Increased serum methaemalbumin (Schumm's test)
   f. Decreased or absent serum haptoglobins
   g. Decreased isotopic (^{51}Cr) red cell survival. Can be combined with organ surface counting to determine sites of red cell destruction. Arrange with the haematology laboratory
   h. Sometimes, low serum folate with megaloblastic changes (p. 17).
2. Indicating increased red cell production:
   a. Hb (is haemolysis compensated or not?)
   b. Increased reticulocyte count, often associated with a moderated increase in MCV (as reticulocytes are larger than normal red cells), polychromasia on the blood film, and nucleated RBC (p. 245)

    c. Increased leucocyte and platelet counts (due to increased haemopoeitic drive)

    d. Erythroid hyperplasia (but bone marrow examination not always necessary).

3. Suggesting cause of the haemolysis:

    a. Red cell clumps on the film or in sample bottle (cold agglutinins (p. 246), often result in false high MCV)

    b. Spherocytes on blood film (hereditary spherocytosis, warm auto-immune haemolytic anaemia)

    c. Red cell fragments, helmet cells (p. 243) (heart valve haemolysis, MAHA)

    d. Heinz bodies (p. 245) (usually found during acute episodes of drug induced haemolysis in G6PD deficiency). Demonstrated by special staining techniques.

GENERAL MANAGEMENT OF HAEMOLYSIS

1. Establish cause and remove if possible.
2. Folic acid: patients with chronic haemolysis, especially if pregnant, can become folate depleted, exacerbating the anaemia. Give 5 mg p.o. daily.
3. Transfusion: may be necessary during acute severe haemolysis, or in pregnancy; with chronic haemolysis transfusion requirements should be gauged by the patients clinical state and not just the Hb level. See specific causes of haemolysis (below) for detailed requirements.

AUTO-IMMUNE HAEMOLYTIC ANAEMIA (AIHA)

Antibody coated red cells are destroyed in the spleen and elsewhere in the reticulo-endothelial system or (rarely) haemolysed in the circulation by a complement fixing antibody. The antibody may have maximal activity at 37°C ('warm' AIHA) or at 4°C ('cold' AIHA).

Warm AIHA

Causes

1. Idiopathic.
2. Secondary to connective tissue diseases e.g. SLE.
3. Secondary to drugs (p. 233).
4. Secondary to B-cell neoplasms (p. 119).

Investigations

1. To establish presence of haemolysis as detailed above.
2. Direct antiglobulin (Coombs) test (DAT) to detect antibody on red cell surface. Usually IgG and/or complement.
3. Bone marrow (to search for underlying lymphoma).
4. ^{51}Cr red cell survival with surface counting over spleen, liver and bone marrow to establish site of red cell destruction.

Treatment

1. General measures as detailed above.
2. Steroids, e.g. prednisolone 40–80 mg daily until response seen (60% respond) then gradually tailed.
3. Splenectomy; consider when:
   a. DAT shows IgG only on red cell surface
   b. Failure of steroid treatment, or unacceptably high dose required
   c. If ^{51}Cr labelling of red cells shows spleen to be a major site of red cell destruction.
4. Other immunosuppressive agents, e.g. azathioprine 2–2.5 mg/kg/day. Causes macrocytosis and requires careful monitoring to prevent marrow suppression.
5. Transfusion: avoid if possible. May be required in severe haemolysis whilst waiting for steroids to work, but cross-matching may be difficult (p. 206).

Cold AIHA

Causes

1. Idiopathic.
2. Secondary to B-cell malignancy e.g. CLL (p. 117).
3. Associated with infections e.g. mycoplasma pneumonia, glandular fever.

Investigations

1. To establish haemolysis as detailed above.
2. Cold agglutinin titre: looking for agglutinating antibodies against adult red cells (anti-I) or cord blood red cells (anti-i). Usually < 1 in 16 in normal, > 1 in 1000 in cold AIHA. Keep specimen at 37°C until serum separated.
3. Mycoplasma antibody titres if history of chest infection. Glandular fever screening test and blood film examination for reactive lymphocytes if history suggestive.
4. DAT, usually complement only on red cells.
5. WBC count and differential.
6. Bone marrow examination and biopsy of any enlarged lymph nodes if underlying lymphoma suspected.
7. Protein electrophoresis (for paraprotein).

Treatment

1. *Keep the patient warm.*
2. General measures as detailed above.
3. Treat cause if not idiopathic.
4. Immunosuppression with chlorambucil 2–6 mg daily (p. 150) in severe cases.
5. Steroids and splenectomy are usually ineffective.
6. Avoid transfusion if possible. If essential use packed cells (contain less complement), an in-line blood warmer and keep the patient warm.

HAEMOLYTIC DISEASE OF THE NEWBORN

Definition

Maternal antibody (usually IgG) in the mother's serum crosses the placenta haemolysing her baby's red cells, causing death in utero or anaemia and jaundice in the neonate.

Causes

1. Anti-D: Rhesus (D) negative mother is immunised against D by a fetal-maternal bleed from her Rhesus (D) positive baby, or more rarely by the inadvertent transfusion of Rh D positive blood. Successive Rhesus positive babies then suffer from haemolysis.
2. Anti-A and anti-B: Group 0 mother (whose serum will always contain IgM anti-A and anti-B which does not cross the placenta) develops haemolytic (IgG) anti-A and/or anti-B which affects her A or B baby.
3. Other antibodies: commonest are anti-c̄, anti-Kell, and other Rhesus and non-Rhesus atypical red-cell antibodies. These may result from immunising blood transfusion or fetal-maternal bleeds.

Prevention of Rhesus (D) haemolytic disease

1. Most immunising fetal-maternal bleeds will occur at delivery, therefore Rhesus (D) negative mothers should receive 500 i.u. of anti-D by i.m. injection within 72 hours of delivery to remove potentially sensitising Rh positive fetal cells. This dose of anti-D will remove 4 ml of packed Rh positive red cells; the fetal cell (Kleihauer) test performed on the mother's blood after delivery will detect larger fetal-maternal bleeds requiring further doses of anti-D.

2. Other potentially traumatic events that may result in fetal-maternal bleeds (e.g. amniocentesis, termination of pregnancy, miscarriage, antepartum haemorrhage, abdominal trauma) should be covered by 50 µg of i.m. anti-D before 20 weeks, and 100 µg after 20 weeks. After 20 weeks a fetal cell test should also be performed.
3. Do not transfuse Rh positive blood to Rh negative women in the reproductive age group. If such transfusion occurs consult with the haematologist regarding the large doses of anti-D that it will be necessary to give to remove the Rh positive red cells.
4. Anti-D sensitisation occurs by small fetal-maternal bleeds during pregnancy and in future administration of anti-D during pregnancy may become standard practice. However, failure to administer anti-D post partum is still a major cause of sensitisation.

Investigations

1. On parents' blood:
   a. Screening tests for atypical red cell antibodies should be performed:
      (i)   At booking in all women
      (ii) In Rh(D) negative women at 20–24 weeks (when amniocentesis may be performed if necessary) and at 36 weeks (when early delivery may be induced if necessary)
      (iii) Ideally at 36 weeks in all women in preparation for possible maternal transfusion at delivery
   b. Women with atypical RBC antibodies at booking will need more frequent testing — consult with haematologist
   c. Genotype husband's red cells to assess likelihood of baby carrying the relevant antigen (e.g. if father is CDe/cde then only half his children will inherit the D antigen and be susceptible).
2. On cord blood:
   a. Direct antiglobulin test, ABO and Rhesus grouping — to determine if baby is affected
   b. Haemoglobin and bilirubin to determine the severity of haemolysis. In a full-term baby, a cord blood haemoglobin < 12 g/dl and/or bilirubin > 80 umol/l are indications for exchange transfusion (see below).

Treatment

1. In pregnancy:
   If strong possibility of affected baby (a rising titre of antibody and previously affected infant are more worrying than the actual titre) consider:
   a. High resolution ultrasound to guide amniocentesis and check for fetal maturity and ascites
   b. Amniocentesis to obtain amniotic fluid for bilirubin estimation — may help predict severity of haemolysis
   c. Early delivery and exchange transfusion if lecithin/sphingomyelin ratio in amniotic fluid suggests adequate fetal lung maturity
   d. If not mature enough for delivery, intrauterine transfusion (at specialist centre)
   e. Maternal plasmapheresis using cell separator to remove anti-D (at specialist centre)
   f. Amnioscopic fetal blood sampling may be the future method of choice for assessing degree of haemolysis and fetal genotype in early pregnancy.
2. At delivery:
   a. Exchange transfusion using fresh (< 24 hours old) O Rhesus negative packed cells, cross-matched against maternal serum
   b. Phototherapy (blue light decomposes bilirubin) and administration of phenobarbitone (to induce liver enzymes) have a small but useful role.

ABO haemolytic disease

Commoner but relatively mild. Investigations and treatment during pregnancy are unnecessary. At delivery treat as above.

ß THALASSAEMIA MAJOR

Clinical features

1. Affects mainly babies of Mediterranean or Indian origin.
2. Both parents will have ß thalassaemia trait (p. 14).
3. Clinically normal at birth (as fetal Hb does not contain ß chains) but may be diagnosed from cord blood in at-risk pregnancy by complete absence of Hb A on electrophoresis and no ß chain synthesis.
4. Progressive anaemia, stunting of growth, jaundice, hepatosplenomegaly in infancy.

Laboratory features

1. Microcytic hypochromic anaemia.
2. Blood film shows nucleated red cells, target cells, polychromasia, punctate basophilia and anisopoikilocytosis.
3. Elevated HbF ($> 50\%$) with variable A_2.
4. Unconjugated hyperbilirubinaemia.
5. Marrow shows erythroid hyperplasia, dyserythropoiesis, and increased iron stores.
6. Marked inbalance in ß and $\propto$ haemoglobin chain synthesis ($\propto$/ß ratio of $> 3:1$).
7. High serum iron, low TIBC, high serum ferritin.

Other investigations

1. X-rays: The chronic marrow hyperplasia results in bossing and 'hair on end' skull X-ray appearances, protruberant maxillae (prognathism) and fractures of phalanges.
2. Endocrine assessment: Iron overload may impair all endocrine organs (e.g. pancreas), discuss with paediatricians.

MANAGEMENT

These children are entirely transfusion dependent.

Before first transfusion

1. Ensure diagnostic investigations (above) have been done — it is very difficult to make a diagnosis after transfusion.
2. Consider active immunisation against hepatitis B.
3. HLA typing of siblings in case marrow transplant is feasible.
4. Suggest parents contact local thalassaemia society.

Hypertransfusion therapy

Aims

1. Avoid symptoms of anaemia — good quality of life.
2. Suppression of marrow hyperplasia, avoiding stunting and bone deformities.
3. Reduce GIT absorption of iron.
4. Prevent hypersplenism.

Method

1. Transfuse every three to six weeks to keep Hb over 11 g/dl and to take Hb level to 15 g/dl with each transfusion.
2. Carefully chart pre-transfusion and post-transfusion Hb — splenectomy may be decided upon by assessment of blood requirements.

Complications
1. Iron overload: without iron chelation therapy (see below) death from iron overload occurs at age 10–20 years even in those patients not hypertransfused.
2. Development of red cell, white cell, platelet and anti-Gm antibodies. May require leucocyte depleted or washed red cells (p. 206).

Iron chelation therapy
1. Desferrioxamine usually started at age two to four years.
2. Maximal urinary iron excretion achieved by using a motorised syringe driver (e.g. Graseby Dynamics MS 18) giving nocturnal 8-hourly infusion into abdominal subcutaneous tissue.
   Dose: 50 mg/kg/night for 5 nights per week, or:
         80 mg/kg/night for 3 nights per week.
3. During blood transfusion also give 6 gm desferrioxamine in 20 ml water for injection and inject piggy-back into drip rubber using syringe driver over eight hours.
4. Vitamin C 200 mg p.o. daily every day of desferrioxamine therapy to help mobilise iron.
5. Assess degree of iron overload periodically (serum ferritin).

Splenectomy
Consider splenectomy if:
1. Blood requirement > 600 ml/kg/year of whole blood, particularly with a spleen > 6 cm below costal margin.
2. Physical discomfort from massive splenomegaly.
3. Neutropenia and/or thrombocytopenia from hypersplenism. See page 94 for complications of splenectomy in children.

HEREDITARY SPHEROCYTOSIS (HS)

An inherited membrane defect rendering the red cells susceptible to destruction in the spleen, and characterised by spherocytes in the blood.

Clinical features

1. Anaemia, jaundice and splenomegaly, usually presenting in childhood. The anaemia may often be compensated.
2. Autosomal dominant inheritance.
3. Commonest in North Europeans.
4. Predisposition to pigment gall stones.
5. Aplastic crises and chronic leg ulcers may be seen (p. 46).

Investigations

1. Numberous spherocytes on blood film.
2. Increased osmotic fragility (Fig. 6.1).
3. Elevated MCHC.
4. Other general laboratory features of haemolysis as detailed above.

Treatment

1. General measures as above.
2. Splenectomy should be performed in all anaemic children and young adults and will almost always result in normal Hb levels, but see precautions regarding splenectomy in children detailed on page 94.

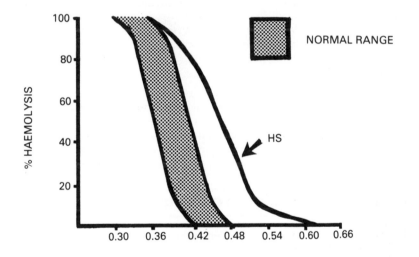

Fig. 6.1 Red cell osmotic fragility curve in a non-splenectomised patient with hereditary spherocytosis (HS). The long 'tail' to the curve is characteristic

GLUCOSE 6-PHOSPHATE DEHYDROGENASE DEFICIENCY (G6PD)

By far the commonest of the red cell enzyme defects, rendering the haemoglobin molecule susceptible to oxidative damage with the formation of Heinz bodies and consequent haemolysis.

Clinical features

1. Haemolytic episodes associated with drugs (p. 235), infections, in the neonatal period, and eating broad beans (favism).
2. X-linked inheritance, but some heterozygous females are affected, and homozygous females are relatively common.
3. Commonest in Mediteranean, Black and Asian races.
4. Haemolysis is usually self-limiting for a particular dose of causative drug as the young reticulocytes have higher G6PD levels.

Investigations

1. Heinz bodies (particles of denatured precipitated haemoglobin) demonstrated in the red cells by special stains during haemolytic episodes.
2. Low red cell G6PD levels. A high reticulocyte count may mask this as young red cells have higher G6PD activity.
3. Other general features of haemolytic anaemia as detailed on page 30.

Treatment

1. Remove or treat cause if possible.
2. General measures in treatment of haemolysis as above.
3. Warn patient to avoid relevant drug or food (p. 236).
4. Transfusion of normal red cells resistant to haemolysis may be necessary in severe haemolysis, or exchange transfusion in neonate.

REFERENCES

Beutler E 1979 Red cell enzyme defects as diseases and non-diseases. Blood 54(1): 1–7
Fraser I D, Tovey G H 1976 Observations on Rhesus isoimmunisation: past, present and future. Clinics in Haematology 5(1): 149–163
Flaherty T, Geary C G 1979 Auto-immune haemolytic anaemia. British Journal of Hospital Medicine 22: 334–345
Weatherall D J, Clegg J B 1981 The thalassaemia syndromes, 3rd edn. Blackwell, Oxford

7. SICKLE CELL SYNDROMES

These include Haemoglobin SS, Haemoglobin SC and Haemoglobin S–ß thalassaemia variants often considered together under the general heading of sickle cell disease (SCD).

CLINICAL FEATURES IN STEADY-STATE SCD

Clinical features of a patient with sickle crisis cannot be usefully interpreted unless they are viewed in the context of abnormalities that may exist in the steady-state of the disease.

1. General
   a. Frequently thinner and shorter than non-sicklers
   b. Mild clinical jaundice
   c. Epistaxis common
   d. Recurrent infections, particularly with capsulate organisms
   e. Leg ulcers, unusual in the UK.
2. Cardiovascular system
   a. Impaired cardiac function secondary to chronic severe anaemia and iron overload in transfused patients
   b. Cardiomegaly with displaced forceful apex beat and parasternal heave. Pansystolic murmur due to anaemia
   c. Chest X-ray shows globular cardiomegaly, prominent pulmonary artery and prominent vascular shadows, even in the absence of pulmonary hypertension.
3. Respiratory system
   a. Repeated pulmonary infection and/or infarction may lead to cor pulmonale and pulmonary hypertension.
4. Gastrointestinal system
   a. Increased incidence of peptic ulceration
   b. Pigment gall-stones common
   j   c. Spleen usually impalpable in adults with Hb SS
   d. Smooth, non-tender hepatomegaly common in adults
   e. Mildly impaired liver function due to intra-hepatic sickling.

40

5. Genitourinary system
   a. Asymptomatic poor concentrating ability
   b. Haematuria common, due to papillary necrosis
   c. Impotence after repeated attacks of priapism
   d. Sub-fertility in males.
6. Central nervous system
   a. Segmental dilatation of retinal veins, most marked in lower temporal regions
   b. Vitreous haemorrhages may occur, sometimes leading to retinal tears
   c. Mild sensori-neural hearing loss common.
7. Musculoskeletal system
   Increased incidence of:
   a. Osteomyelitis
   b. Septic arthritis
   c. Gout
   d. Aseptic necrosis of hip or shoulder, particularly in Hb SC disease.

LABORATORY FEATURES IN STEADY-STATE SCD

1. Haemoglobin 5–10g/dl (Hb SS), 9–11g/dl (Hb SC or Hb S-ßthal$^+$). Normochromic, normocytic anaemia, except in Hb S ß-thal$^+$ when microcytic.
2. Blood film: variable numbers of irreversibly sickled cells. Marked poikilocytosis. Target cells (particularly in Hb SC). Variable numbers of nucleated red cells. Red cell inclusions such as Howell-Jolly bodies, basophilic stippling.
3. Mild neutrophilia, $12–20 \times 10^9/1$ common, with left shift.
4. Platelet count normal or raised in Hb SS, normal in Hb SC. A low platelet count suggests hypersplenism.
5. Reticulocytes 10–25%.
6. Uric acid raised in adults.
7. Bilirubin usually 20–60 mmol/l.
8. Mild elevation of LDH and AST common.
9. Low plasma urea.

VASO-OCCLUSIVE CRISES

Sickle cell crisis, known as 'painful' or 'vaso-occlusive crisis' is a syndrome of generalised or localised pain due to vaso-occlusion by sickled red cells. Sickle crisis can be seen in any patient with sickle cell variants Haemoglobin SS, Haemoglobin SC or Haemoglobin S-ß-thalassaemia. Crises are seen in individuals with sickle trait (AS) only in very exceptional circumstances.

Known provoking factors

1. Recent hypoxia — inadequate oxygenation during or immediately after general anaesthetic, air travel.
2. Dehydration, including alcohol excess.
3. Infections. Any organism, including malaria.
4. Pregnancy. Especially last trimester and immediately post-partum.
5. Exposure to cold.
6. Metabolic acidosis after intense exercise.

General management of all vaso-occlusive crises

Aims of treatment: to treat underlying cause, prevent extension of vaso-occlusion, relieve pain, prevent complications.

1. Bed rest.
2. Keep patient warm.
3. Close medical and nursing observation.
4. Arrange baseline investigations: Hb, WBC, platelet count, reticulocyte count, blood group and save serum, urea and electrolytes, liver function tests, chest X-ray.
5. Immediate and adequate analgesia. Discuss with the patient what they feel they need. Pain is totally subjective and the doctor cannot assess the distress it is causing the patient. Analgesic abuse in Sicklers in the UK is virtually unknown. Adequate analgesia will vary from paracetamol to DF118 to oral pethidine to intramuscular pethidine, even hourly. Occasionally morphine is required. While the pain is severe, write up the dose for regular administration and discuss your treatment with the nursing staff who may rightly be reluctant to give large doses of regular analgesia unless you make it clear that that is what is needed. Review the need for analgesia, with the patient, at least once daily. Aspirin or one of the non-steroidal anti-inflammatory drugs are often useful for bone pain. Mild sedation, e.g. with 2 mg diazepam t.d.s., may sometimes be helpful.
6. Search for and treat underlying infection
   a. Arrange MSU, blood cultures, throat swab, sputum culture (if present) save acute serum for viral serology, mycoplasma CFT, blood for pneumococcal antigen
   b. After cultures taken, start appropriate wide-spectrum antibiotic active against capsulate organisms, e.g. amoxycillin 500 mg t.d.s. orally. Change the antibiotic as dictated by new clinical or microbiological findings.

7. Rehydration. This is vital
   a. In milder crises, fluids can be given by mouth to preserve the veins but this requires a great deal of patient effort and nursing supervision
   b. In severe crises, set up an intravenous infusion of 50–80 ml/kg body weight/24 hours; adjust for cardiovascular status. Use any of: normal saline, dextrose-saline or 5% dextrose. Add potassium supplementation as needed.
8. Oxygen therapy is generally unhelpful unless the patient is actually hypoxic. If you suspect this, prove it by taking arterial blood gases.
9. In severe crises, the only definitive treatment, if there is no response to general measures, is exchange blood transfusion to reduce the level of Hb S to less than 30%. The indications for exchange are discussed later.
10. Fever, tachycardia and sometimes hypotension can often be seen in vaso-occlusive crises without infection being present.

Bone/joint vaso-occlusive crises

1. Usually presents with severe, constant, deep-seated pain in one or more sites. There is often a prodomal history of a few days intermittent mild pain at the same site.
2. On examination, there may or may not be tenderness over the site and the affected site may be warm. Look for joint effusions.
3. Repeated involvement of the same site suggests avascular necrosis or osteomyelitis. Occasionally, severe bone sickling may cause a spontaneous fracture.
4. Differential diagnosis includes gout, osteomyelitis, and rheumatic fever. X-ray of the affected area and bone scan may be very helpful.

Abdominal vaso-occlusive crises

1. Presents with constant, severe pain all over abdomen. May be accompanied by nausea or vomiting.
2. On examination, the abdomen will be tender, sometimes with rebound tenderness. There may be abdominal distension and reduced or absent bowel sounds.
3. Arrange for erect and supine abdominal X-rays to look for fluid levels and air under the diaphragm.
4. Take regular girth measurements; increase suggests mesenteric infarction or hyper-sequestration in liver/spleen.
5. Take blood for serum amylase.
6. Treat severe cases with nil by mouth and gastric suction progressing to fluids only as the signs resolve.
7. Differential diagnosis includes splenic infarction (pleuritic pain in left hypochondrium sometimes associated with shoulder-tip pain and a rub), hepatic infarction, acute pancreatitis, cholecystitis, biliary colic, peptic ulcer disease or unconnected surgical disorders.

Chest syndrome

1. Potentially fatal syndrome of extensive uni- or bi-lateral lung consolidation. Often unproven as to whether it is primarily infective or infarctive.
2. Presents with pain in back, ribs or 'deep in lungs'. May be pleuritic in nature. Accompanied by dyspnoea, tachypnoea and sometimes cough.
3. Clinical and radiological findings may demonstrate consolidation with or without effusion. Upper lobe vascular diversion is a frequent early sign.
4. Serial arterial blood gas estimations are vital. Lung scan is sometimes helpful and angiography is contra-indicated.
5. Look for fat globules in sputum (derived from embolus of infarcted marrow).
6. Treat hypoxia with oxygen.
7. Arrange chest physiotherapy.

Priapism

1. Priapism is prolonged painful erection of the penis in the absence of sexual or mechanical stimulation. Due to the embarrassing nature of this type of vaso-occlusive crisis, the patient often presents very late. Life-long impotence may be the result.
2. Educate all male sicklers at your clinic to come to the hospital as early as possible in an episode of priapism. There is often a history of recent stuttering priapism with transient nocturnal attacks lasting for 1 to 4 hours.
3. General measures include encouraging micturition and defaecation, short period of brisk exercise, cold baths, local ice packs. Liaise early with genito-urinary surgeons.
4. If no response, arrange urgent exchange transfusion and proceed to surgery, ideally done with spinal anaesthesia. Initial surgical procedure is usually direct aspiration of the corpora cavernosa. If this does not relieve the priapism, more definitive surgical procedures such as cavernosum-spongiosum shunt may be necessary.

CNS vaso-occlusion

1. Take any CNS symptom or sign extremely seriously.
2. If CNS signs are established arrange for urgent cerebral computerised axial tomography scan.
3. In severe or worsening neurological deficit proceed immediately to exchange transfusion.

Exchange transfusion

1. Indications (controversial)
   a. CNS sickling
   b. Severe chest syndrome or abdominal crisis that does not respond to general measures within twelve hours, or is showing signs of deteriorating before that time
   c. Priapism that does not respond within hours or permanent impotence may result
   d. As a planned procedure before major surgery and in pregnancy
   e. As prophylaxis in a patient with frequent severe painful crises.
2. Problems
   a. Individuals with Hb SS are very active producers of transfusion allo-antibodies. An individual may develop so many antibodies after one or more exchanges that it proves almost impossible to find compatible blood for them subsequently. Some centres transfuse blood of the same full Rhesus and Kell phenotype as the recipient in an effort to delay the development of allo-antibodies
   b. Venous access. Ideally two good venepunctures are required with cannulae or butterfly needles of at least 21 gauge, though a single needle may be used to both take and give blood (see p. 254).

      Blood in SCD is hyperviscous and will often need to be aspirated with a 60 ml syringe as it may clot in the tubing if allowed to drain without suction
   c. It is usually necessary to reduce the percentage of Hb S in the blood to 20–30%. This may require exchange of 1–2 total blood volumes. Hence any of the complications of massive transfusion (see Ch. 30) may ensue.

Prevention of vaso-occlusive crises

1. Education of the patient and his/her family
   a. Early hospital visits if unwell
   b. Avoid getting chilled
   c. Take extra fluid in hot weather or during unusual exercise. Avoid excess alcohol
   d. At first signs of pain, rest in bed and take at least two cups of fluid hourly during waking hours
   e. Attend clinic at least yearly so that their steady-state pattern can be observed by their doctors.

2. Prophylaxis against infection
    a. Full immunization programme, including pneumococcal vaccine
    b. Anti-malarial prophylaxis if in endemic area
    c. Prophylactic penicillin V 250 mg b.d. from 6 months old to at least school leaving age
    d. Prophylactic antibiotics e.g. ampicillin plus metronidazole, for surgical procedures.

Sudden increase in degree of anaemia

The red cell parameters in sickle vaso-occlusive crisis are usually unchanged from the steady-state. Patients with SCD may also suddenly become more anaemic than usual with a painless drop in the haemoglobin to more than 2 g/dl below the steady state level. This can be due to:

1. Aplastic crisis
    a. Presents with weakness, listlessness, shortness of breath, often of acute onset
    b. Most common in childhood and early teens
    c. May be preceding history of drugs, excess alcohol, viral illness in the patient or in a close contact
    d. Haemoglobin lower than usual and reticulocytes low or even absent
    e. Take blood for folic acid estimation, cross-match, viral serology (particularly parvo virus and Paul-Bunnell) and search for other evidence of infection
    f. If not severe, observe only. The episode is usually self-limiting, lasting 5–10 days
    g. If the drop in haemoglobin is severe and symptomatic then give blood transfusion.
2. Reticulo-endothelial sequestration
    a. Usually in children aged 6 months to 3 years with Hb SS and Hb S-ß-thal disease. Occasionally seen in pregnant women with Hb SC
    b. Extremely rapid, profound fall in haemoglobin to 3 g/dl or less with an increase in the reticuloyte count
    c. Provokes circulatory failure with hypovolaemic shock within a few hours
    d. Associated with sudden splenic enlargement with severe abdominal pain. The patient is very pale, hypotensive and has a rigid distended abdomen
    e. Rapid blood transfusion, uncrossmatched if the situation is desperate, will be life-saving.

3. Folate deficiency (p. 17).
4. Other causes.
   Do not forget that patients with SCD may become more anaemic than usual for reasons unconnected with their disease, e.g. blood-loss, GGPD deficiency.

REFERENCES

Charache S 1981 Treatment of sickle cell anaemia. Annual review of Medicine 32: 195–206
Fleming A F 1982 Sickle cell disease. Churchill Livingstone, Edinburgh Luzzatto L 1981 Sickle cell anaemia in tropical Africa. Clinics in Haematology 10(3): 757–784

Part 2
EXCESS OF BLOOD CELLS

8. THROMBOCYTOSIS

DEFINITION

A rise in the blood platelet count to over $400 \times 10^9/l$.

CAUSES

Primary — myeloproliferative disorders

1. Essential thrombocythaemia (see below).
2. Myelofibrosis (30% of cases have thrombocytosis) (p. 27).
3. Chronic granulocytic leukaemia (p. 111).
4. Polycythaemia rubra vera (p. 60).

Secondary

1. Physiological
   a. Vigorous exercise
   b. Childbirth
2. Reactive
   a. Following acute and chronic haemorrhage
   b. After trauma and operation (starts rising to 35–150% above normal after sixth post-operative day, usually normal by 16 days)
   c. Acute and chronic infections (e.g. TB, osteomyelitis)
   d. Chronic inflammation e.g. sarcoidosis, collagen disorders, ulcerative colitis, Crohn's disease
   e. Rebound on recovery of thrombocytopenia or generalised marrow hypoplasia (e.g. after cytotoxics)
   f. Post splenectomy (often rises to $1000 \times 10^9/l$, maximal at 12th day, and falls slowly towards normal over next two months) and splenic vein thrombosis

g. Accompanying haemolysis
h. Malignant disease e.g. carcinoma, lymphoma
i. Iron deficiency anaemia.

In at least 90% of cases, the cause of the thrombocytosis is self evident and can safely be ignored unless there are other predisposing factors for thromboembolism (p. 178) in which case treatment with aspirin or dipyridamole may be used (p. 187). Assessment of the other 10% of cases where a diagnosis is not obvious involves:

1. A systematic search for underlying disease.
2. Establishing a diagnosis of essential thrombocythaemia (see below).

Clinical features
A secondary thrombocytosis is generally asymptomatic except for symptoms of the underlying disease, or thromboembolism (p. 180).

Laboratory features
A high platelet count from any cause may cause falsely high results for serum potassium, uric acid, calcium, phosphate, zinc and lactic dehydrogenase.

PRIMARY (ESSENTIAL) THROMBOCYTHAEMIA

Clinical features

1. Bleeding:
    a. Epistaxes and recurrent gastro-intestinal haemorrhage
    b. Bruising common, petechiae rare
    c. Rarely, massive haemorrhage with trauma or surgery.
2. Thromboembolism:
    a. DVT and pulmonary embolism common
    b. May be unusual sites e.g. mesenteric vessels, dorsal vein of penis, gangrene of toes, splenic vein thrombosis
    c. May present as odd neurological abnormalities e.g. amaurosis fugax, vertigo, confusion, transient ischaemic attacks. Full neurological assessment is important.
3. Peptic ulcer disease common.
4. Organomegaly
    a. Splenomegaly common, from just tippable to 10 cm enlarged. Splenic atrophy may also be seen due to recurrent splenic infarcts
    b. Moderate hepatomegaly common.
    c. Lymphadenopathy very unusual.
5. Symptoms and signs of secondary hyperuricaemia.

Laboratory features

1. Blood count and film
   a. Platelet count usually $> 1000 \times 10^9/1$ (a sudden increase in an already high platelet count may be due to splenic vein thrombosis)
   b. Platelet size and shape abnormal — giant platelets
   c. Red cells may show hyposplenic features (burr cells, spherocytes, target cells, Howell-Jolly bodies)
   d. Slightly raised red cell count in 30% (differential diagnosis with polycythaemia rubra vera may be difficult)
   e. Often neutrophilia with shift to the left. A slight increase in basophils and eosinophils common
   f. NAP score increased
   g. Hypochromic microcytic anaemia common (due to chronic occult blood loss).
2. Bone marrow (aspirate and trephine biopsy needed)
   a. Marked increased in number and size of megakaryocytes
   b. May be increased numbers of white cell and red cell precursors
   c. Chromosome abnormalities quite common
   d. Biopsy often shows increased reticulin.
3. Platelet function tests may show abnormal aggregation responses including spontaneous aggregation.
4. Serum B12 and uric acid usually raised.

Treatment

1. Urgent reduction in massive platelet count in severe haemorrhage or before emergency surgery: referral to a specialist unit for thrombocytapheresis on a cell separator or start oral hydroxyurea at a dose of 2–5 g daily.

Table 8.1 Differentiating between 1° and 2° thrombocytosis

	1° thrombocythaemia	2° thrombocytosis
Platelet morphology	Abnormal	Usually normal
Platelet function tests	Abnormal	Usually normal
Bleeding time	Usually prolonged	Usually normal
Basophil leucocytosis	Usually present	Absent
Platelet count	Usually $< 1000 \times 10^9/1$	Usually $< 1000 \times 10^9/1$
Clinical splenomegaly	Present in 30%	Absent*
Duration	Persistent	Often transient
Thromboembolism/haemorrhage	Common	Unusual
Age	Usually > 60 years	Any age

*Unless abnormal due to underlying disease

2. Reducing the megakaryocyte mass: single injection of radio-active phosphorous (^{32}P) or use hydroxyurea or busulphan as in CGL (p. 114). Both take two to six weeks before exerting any therapeutic effect.
3. Preventing platelet aggregation: aspirin 300 mg twice-weekly, dipyridamole 100–300 mg daily.
4. Treatment of established thromboembolism: use usual protocol of heparin and warfarin (p. 183) but unusually high doses of heparin may be needed (because of anti-heparin effect of platelets).
5. Prophylactic anti-coagulants: probably of little use except that subcutaneous heparin may be used in peri-operative patients.
6. Splenectomy: of no value except in the rare cases complicated by myelofibrosis and hypersplenism, and may exacerbate thrombocytosis.

REFERENCES

Murphy S 1983 Thrombocytosis and thrombocythaemia. Clinics in Haematology 12(1): 89–106
Ozer F L, Truax W E, Miesch D C, Levin W C 1960 Primary haemorrhagic thrombocythaemia. American Journal of Medicine 28: 807–823

9. LEUCOCYTOSIS

DEFINITION

A raised total white cell count, over $11 \times 10^9/1$. This can be due to an absolute increase in one or more of the different types of white cells (most commonly a neutrophil leucocytosis) and diagnostic investigations depend on which white cell type is involved.

Leukaemoid reaction

Occasionally, the leucocytosis is so marked that it mimics the blood findings found in leukaemia and it is then referred to as a leukaemoid reaction. There is no single accepted definition of a leukaemoid reaction but it usually refers to a leucocyte count of more than $50 \times 10^9/1$ in a patient in whom the subsequent clinical course or post-mortem findings do not confirm the diagnosis of leukaemia.

Commonest causes of leukaemoid reaction
1. Mimicking chronic granulocytic leukaemia (see Table 9.1).
2. Mimicking chronic lymphatic leukaemia:
    a. Pertussis (whooping-cough) infection.
3. Mimicking acute lymphoblastic leukaemia:
    a. Infectious monucleosis
    b. Circulating neuroblastoma tumour cells.

NEUTROPHIL LEUCOCYTOSIS (NEUTROPHILIA)

Causes

1. Physiological
    a. Pregnancy
    b. Strenuous exercise
    c. In neonates
    d. After adrenaline or corticosteroid therapy.

55

Table 9.1   Differential diagnosis of neutrophil leukaemoid reaction and chronic granulocytic leukaemia

	Leukaemoid reaction	C G L
WBC count	Usually < 100 x 10⁹/1	Often > 100 x 10⁹/1
White cell morphology	Mature neutrophils with left shift to band forms. Few metamyelocytes and myelocytes	Mature neutrophils and myelocytes are predominant cells. Metamyelocytes uncommon. Occasional promyelocytes and blasts
Neutrophil granulation	Toxic granulation in neutrophils	Granulation in neutrophils normal or hypogranular
Neutrophil alkaline phosphatase score	Usually high	Usually low
Splenomegaly	None	Present
Haemoglobin	Usually normal	Often moderately low
Platelet count	Normal/slightly raised	May be > 1000 x 10⁹/1
Marrow cytogenetics	Normal	Philadelphia chromosome usually present

2. Acute infections
Usually generalised, sometimes localized
  a. Most commonly bacterial infections due to cocci
  b. Others: bacterial baccilli, some viruses, parasites.
3. Tissue damage
  a. Inflammatory diseases, including
    (i) Collagen disorders
    (ii) Crohn's disease, ulcerative colitis
    (iii) Gout
  b. Tissue necrosis, including
    (i) After surgery
    (ii) Myocardial infarction
    (iii) Non-infected gangrene
    (iv) Tissue bleed e.g. haemarthrosis, sub-arachnoid haemorrhage
    (v) Crush injuries, burns
    (vi) Intestinal obstruction
  c. Underlying malignant disease, particularly with metastases
  d. Any allergic reactions, particularly anaphylaxis (an eosinophilia (see below) is also often present)
  e. Metabolic
    (i) Circulatory arrest
    (ii) Diabetic ketoacidosis
    (iii) Pre-eclampsia
    (iv) Profound uraemia
    (v) Poisoning with chemicals, drugs or venoms
  f. As part of increased marrow response
    (i) Haemorrhage
    (ii) Haemolysis

    g. Primary myeloproliferative disorder (a basophilia is also often present)
- (i)   Chronic granulocytic leukaemia
- (ii) Primary thrombocythaemia
- (iii) Polycythaemia rubra vera
- (iv) Myelofibrosis

    h. After therapeutic immunisation.

Investigation

History and examination will usually reveal the cause. If not immediately apparent:

1. Full bacteriological screen including MSU, appropriate swabs, Mantoux test.
2. Auto-antibody screen and rheumatoid factor.
3. Haematological tests (see Table 9.1).

EOSINOPHIL LEUCOCYTOSIS (EOSINOPHILIA)

Causes

1. Allergic disorders including asthma, hay fever, drug hypersensitivity, urticaria.
2. Skin diseases particularly pemphigus, dermatitis herpetiformis.
3. Parasitic infection including trichinosis, schistosomiasis, hookworm, ascaris.
4. Collagen disorders.
5. Lymphoma, especially disseminated Hodgkins disease.
6. Malignant disease of any type.
7. Myeloproliferative disorders, especially CGL.
8. Tropical eosinophilia, Loeffler's syndrome. Associated with respiratory symptoms and pulmonary infiltrates.
9. Hypereosinophilia syndrome. A diagnosis made when no underlying cause for a prolonged, often massive, eosinophilia is found. A wide spectrum of clinical features is found including fever, rashes, splenomegaly, pulmonary abnormalities and myocardial infiltration.
10. Eosinophilic leukaemia (very rare).

Investigations

The cause is usually obvious from the history and examination, particularly if a careful drug history is taken.

1. Fresh faecal specimen for ova and parasites.
2. Chest X-ray.
3. Rheumatoid factor and anti-nuclear factor.
4. Further tests according to clinical suspicion e.g. skin biopsy, patch test, pulmonary function tests.

BASOPHIL LEUCOCYTOSIS (BASOPHILIA)

Basophil leucocytosis is rare.

Causes

1. Myeloproliferative disorders (see *neutrophil leucocytosis* above).
2. Hypersensitivity reactions, e.g. asthma, anaphylaxis.
3. Recovery phase of acute infection or inflammation.
4. Occasionally seen: lymphoma, smallpox, myxoedema, chicken pox.

MONOCYTOSIS (see Table 9.2)

Causes

1. Chronic bacterial infections e.g. SBE, TB, brucellosis.
2. Temporary phenomenon during early phase of recovery after marrow suppression, e.g. after cytotoxic drug therapy.
3. Primary haematological disease e.g. acute monocytic leukaemia (AML, M4 or M5) chronic myelo-monocytic leukaemia (CMML).
4. Protozoal and rickettsial infections e.g. malaria, kala-azar, Rocky Mountain spotted fever, typhus.
5. Occasionally in collagen disorders, sarcoidosis, Crohn's disease, ulcerative colitis, idiopathic thrombocytopenic purpura.
6. Occasionally in Hodgkins disease and non-Hodgkins lymphomas.
7. In congenital neutropenias, probably as a compensatory phenomenon.

Table 9.2   Differential diagnosis of benign secondary monocytosis from acute monocytic leukaemia and chronic myelomonocytic leukaemia

	Monocytosis	Acute monocytic leukaemia	Chronic myelo-monocytic leukaemia
Age	Any	Peak 40-50 years	Over 50 years
Lymphadenopathy	No	Very common	Common
Gum hypertrophy and skin infiltration	No	Common	No
Splenomegaly	No	Very common	Common
Monocyte morphology	Normal cells	Primitive cells	Atypical mature cells
Haemoglobin and platelet count	Normal	Often very low	Normal or mildly reduced
Blasts in bone marrow	Normal numbers	More than 50%	Less than 30%

LYMPHOCYTOSIS

An increase in the total number of lymphocytes in the peripheral blood. Normal in childhood.

Causes

    a. Normal morphology
       (i)   Chronic lymphocytic leukaemia. The commonest cause of a lymphocytosis in middle-aged and elderly persons
      (ii) Acute infectious lymphocytosis of childhood
     (iii) Whooping cough (pertussis)
     (iv) Some chronic infections e.g. brucellosis, TB, $2°$ syphilis
      (v) Recovery from viral exanthems
     (vi) Rarely, underlying malignancy.
    b. Abnormal morphology
       (i)   Some acute infections e.g. infectious mononucleosis, cytomegalovirus, toxoplasmosis, hepatitis A
      (ii) Acute lymphoblastic leukaemia. The majority of cells will be blasts, but also an excess of lymphocytes
     (iii) Lymphoma, especially lymphosarcoma and Waldenstrom's macroglobulinaemia.

Relative lymphocytosis

An increase in the percentage of lymphocytes, often due to a concomittant decrease in absolute numbers of neutrophils.

Causes
    a. Most conditions associated with neutropenia (p.   ).
    b. Not infrequently in normal healthy individuals, particularly of Negro origin.

REFERENCES

Fredricks R E, Moloney W C 1959 The basophilic granulocyte. Blood 14: 571–576
Maldonado J E 1965 Monocytosis: A current appraisal. Proceedings of the Mayo Clinic 40(3): 248–259

10. POLYCYTHAEMIA

DEFINITION

A raised red cell count almost invariably accompanied by an increased haemoglobin and PCV due to either an increased red cell mass or to a decreased plasma volume.

CLASSIFICATION

Primary

Primary myeloproliferative disease with normal or low erythropoietin levels.

Secondary

Erythropoietin levels raised.
1. As an appropriate response to hyposcia:
    a. Chronic hypoxic pulmonary disease
    b. Congenital heart disease with right to left shunt
    c. Heavy smoking particularly with inhalation
    d. High affinity haemoglobins (rare)
    e. High altitudes.
2. Inappropriate production:
    a. *Renal disease*
       Carcinoma
       Cysts
       Hydronephrosis.
    b. *Tumours*
       Renal
       Hepatic
       Cerebellar
       Uterine.

Relative

Normal red cell mass, reduced plasma volume, erythropoietin levels normal.
    a. Stress or spurious polycythaemia.
    b. Associated with excessive fluid or plasma loss; e.g. diarrhoea, vomiting, pyrexia, excessive diuretics.

CLINICAL FEATURES

Can present as an incidental finding or with symptoms of associated complications or diseases:

General features of primary and secondary polycythaemia

1. Thrombotic disease, particularly CVAs.
2. Headaches and dizzyness.
3. Lethargy and weakness.
4. Visual disturbances.
5. Sweating.
6. Weight loss.
7. Plethoric appearance.
8. Engorged fundal veins.
9. Hypertension.

Features usually seen only in primary polycythaemia rubra vera

1. Gout (due to increased cell turnover).
2. Peptic ulceration.
3. Bleeding — especially GIT.
4. Pruritis — especially after hot bath.
5. Splenomegaly (found in about 75% of patients with PRV).
6. Hepatomegaly.

INVESTIGATIONS

1. Hb, PCV, and RBC. Should be raised on at least two occasions before more extensive investigations are undertaken.
2. WBC and platelet counts.
3. Isotopic estimation of red cell mass and plasma volume. Arrange with haematology laboratory. Essential investigation.
4. Neutrophil alkaline phosphatase (NAP) score. Arrange with haematology laboratory.
5. Uric acid.

6. Iron and total iron binding capacity and serum ferritin (if available), as chronic GIT bleeding often leads to iron deficiency.
7. Serum B12. Raised levels can indicate increased granulopoiesis that is often a feature of PRV.
8. Bone marrow and biopsy to assess cellularity and marrow fibrosis.
9. Arterial oxygen saturation (+/− CXR and pulmonary function tests) to exclude polycythaemia secondary to chronic hypoxic lung disease.
10. Urine microscopy, renal ultrasound or IVP — to exclude renal lesions.
11. LDH — usually normal in contrast to other myeloproliferative diseases such as myelofibrosis where greatly elevated levels can be found.
12. Oxygen dissociation curve to exclude high affinity haemoglobins, when there is a family history of polycythaemia. Usually only carried out by specialist laboratories.
13. Urine erythropoietin. Only available at specialist centres.

ESTABLISHING CAUSE OF POLYCYTHAEMIA

PRV

1. Raised red cell mass (> 36 ml/kg in males and > 32 ml/kg in females).
2. Splenomegaly.
3. Arterial oxygen saturation > 92% (need to correct for PCV).
4. Increased WBC (> $12 \times 10^9/1$) and platelet (> $400 \times 10^9/1$) counts.
5. LAP score > 100.
6. Raised serum B12 (> 900 pg/ml).
7. Bone marrow hypercellularity with increased megakaryocytes +/− increased fibrosis.

Secondary polycythaemia

1. Raised red cell mass (see above).
2. Primary cause detectable:
   a. Pulmonary disease with arterial oxygen saturation < 92%
   b. Heart disease with right to left shunt
   c. Abnormal IVP
   d. Primary tumour
   e. Abnormal haemoglobin.
3. No splenomegaly.
4. Normal WBC and platelet counts, and LAP score.

Relative polycythaemia

1. Stress or spurious:
   Type I — Associated with high normal red cell mass and low normal plasma volume. No features of PRV or evidence of a primary cause. Probably normal variation.
   Type II — Normal red cell mass, but decreased plasma volume. Often associated mild hypertension, and is commonest in obese, stressed males who smoke.
2. When associated with excessive fluid or plasma loss, cause usually clear from the clinical situation.

MANAGEMENT

PRV

Aim is to keep PCV < 45%.

1. Venesection alone or combined with either ^{32}P or chemotheraphy.
2. Radioactive phosphorus (^{32}P) given intravenously. Usual dose is 4–7mCi. Nadir of WBC and platelet counts is at 3–5 weeks, and of RBC count 6–8 weeks. Can be repeated as necessary.
3. Chemotherapy. Usually with alkylating agents such as busulphan 2–6 mg p.o. daily (p. 149), (usually weekly counts for first six weeks), but particularly careful haematological monitoring is necessary to avoid serious bone marrow suppression.

   Approximately 10% of patients with PRV transform to acute myeloid leukaemia, and in many myelofibrosis supervenes. Leukaemic transformation may be commoner in those patients treated with alkylating agents. Average survival is 13–16 years, but may be shorter in those treated with venesection alone.

Secondary polycythaemia

1. Treat any primary cause if possible (e.g. removal of tumour).
2. In patients with pulmonary or cardiovascular disease there is a balance between the beneficial effects of an increased red cell count increasing oxygen delivery to the tissues, and the potentially unwanted effects of increased blood viscosity. Each patient probably has an optimum PCV, and judicious venesection with careful monitoring of the clinical state can be helpful in selected patients in maintaining this optimum level.

Relative polycythaemia

1. Type I — No treatment necessary.
2. Type II — Is associated with a higher than normal incidence of cerebro and cardiovascular events, especially if there is associated hypertension. Although lowering the PCV appears of little benefit, control of hypertension, even if mild, is beneficial and stopping smoking and decreasing weight is to be encouraged. There is currently no satisfactory therapy that will permanently restore the plasma volume to normal in these patients.

REFERENCES

Erslev A J, Caro J 1983 Pathophysiology and classification of Polycythaemia. Scandinavian Journal of Haematology 31: 287–292
Lewis S M 1976 Polycythaemia vera. British Journal of Hospital Medicine 16: 125–132

Part 3
DEFICIENCY OF BLOOD CELLS

11. THROMBOCYTOPENIA

DEFINITION

A platelet count less than $150 \times 10^9/1$. May be due to:
1. Failure of platelet production.
2. Increased rate of removal from the circulation.
3. Combination of both.

CLINICAL FEATURES

1. Prolonged bleeding following injury.
2. Spontaneous bleeding. Unusual with platelet count $> 50 \times 10^9/1$ and common with count $< 20 \times 10^9/1$. Can occur at higher counts if there is associated platelet function defect e.g. myeloproliferative disease.
3. Petechiae. Especially legs, flexures and pressure points.
4. Multiple small bruises.
5. Mucous membrane bleeding, especially from nose.
6. Menorrhagia.
7. Conjunctival and retinal haemorrhage with severe cases.
8. Bleeding from venepuncture and injection sites.
9. Intracranial haemorrhage.

CAUSES

Failure of platelet production

Bone marrow shows decreased or absent megakaryocytes and/or features of any associated condition.
1. Drugs: e.g. chloramphenicol, sulphonamides, phenylbutazone, anticonvulsants, thiazides, cimetidine (p. 238).
2. Virus infections.
3. Megaloblastic anaemia.
4. Malignant infiltration of marrow.

67

5. Leukaemia.
6. Myelofibrosis.
7. Myelodysplastic syndromes.
8. Alcohol.
9. Hypoplastic anaemia.
10. Hereditary.

Increased rate of removal from circulation

Bone marrow shows increased megakaryocytes, and is otherwise usually normal.

Immune

1. Primary — idiopathic thrombocytopenic purpura (ITP).
2. Secondary
   a. Drugs: e.g. quinidine, quinine, gold, sulphonamides
   b. Other diseases: e.g. SLE, CLL, lymphomas, viral infections, malaria
   c. Miscellaneous: e.g. post transfusion purpura, neonatal isoimmune thrombocytopenia.

Non immune

Associated with excessive platelet consumption in coagulation. e.g. DIC (see p. 175). TTP (thrombotic thrombocytopenic purpura) syndrome of fever, CNS dysfunction, anaemia and uraemia.

Loss of platelets from systemic circulation

1. Splenomegaly (see p. 91).
2. Cardiopulmonary bypass.
3. Dilution from massive blood transfusion.

THROMBOCYTOPENIA IN VARIOUS AGE GROUPS

Neonate

1. Intrauterine infection:
   Rubella/CMV/toxoplasmosis/syphilis
   May be associated congenital abnormalities.
2. Immune:
   a. Maternal ITP or SLE. Maternal antibodies cross the placenta. Usually self limiting. May need exchange transfusion to decrease antibody levels
   b. Isoimmune. Similar to haemolytic disease of the newborn in that a mother lacking the PLA[1] platelet antigen is sensitised by a PLA[1] positive foetus. The infant may be given PLA[1] negative platelets.

3. DIC:
   Usually associated with seriously ill infants. Resuscitation and treatment of underlying cause most important. May need replacement therapy (see p. 176).
4. Hereditary:
   Rare.

Childhood

1. ITP:
   Commonest cause of thrombocytopenia in childhood.
   Often acute following a viral infection
   Platelet count usually $< 20 \times 10^9/1$
   Spontaneous remission in $> 80\%$ within a few weeks
   Serious intracranial haemorrhage very rare ($< 1\%$)
   Most need no treatment.
2. Viral infections:
   Suppress bone marrow production and cause peripheral platelet destruction.
3. Associated with bone marrow disease:
   Aplasia and leukaemia
   Diagnosis revealed by marrow aspiration and biopsy.
4. Haemolytic-Uraemic Syndrome:
   Microangiopathic haemolytic anaemia (p. 243) (usually numerous fragmented RBC's on blood film), acute renal failure.
   Most important aspect of treatment is management of the renal failure.

Adults

1. ITP:
   Usually insidious onset
   No obvious precipitating cause
   Platelet count often $> 20 \times 10^9/1$
   Chronic course with remissions and relapses
   Spontaneous remissions $< 20\%$
   Asymptomatic patients with platelets $> 50 \times 10^9/1$ should be observed only
   Symptomatic patients may be treated by:
   a. Steroids e.g. prednisone $\geqslant$ 1mg/kg daily
   b. If no response after one month or unacceptably high maintenance dose required, consider splenectomy, further immunosuppression or high dose intravenous IgG — consult with haematologist.
2. Other immune disorders:
   e.g. SLE and CLL.
3. Drugs:
   See above.

4. Bone marrow disease:
   e.g. aplasia, leukaemia, myeloma, myelofibrosis.
5. TTP:
   See above. Plasma exchange and FFP infusions mainstay of treatment.
6. DIC.
7. Splenomegaly.
   See page 91.
8. Post transfusion:
   a. Due to immune platelet destruction, usually occurring about one week following blood transfusion
      Platelet infusions of little use though plasma exchange may help
   b. Dilution due to massive, rapid transfusion.

CLINICAL ASSESSMENT

1. Assess extent and severity of bleeding (oral and fundal haemorrhage often proceeds a cerebral bleed).
2. Enquire about recent viral infections (often associated with acute ITP in children).
3. Take a drug history.
4. Recent transfusion history (immune thrombocytopenia can occur about one week following a transfusion).
5. Any relevant medical history: e.g. SLE, CLL, lymphoma, leukaemia.
6. Any condition present associated with DIC (see p. 175).
7. In neonate, history of sepsis or maternal thrombocytopenia.
8. Examine for splenomegaly.

LABORATORY ASSESSMENT

1. Blood count and film:
   Anaemia and many fragmented cells may suggest DIC, ITP or the haemolytic-uraemic syndrome (see below), or may give evidence of marrow disease (e.g. blast cells).
2. Re-check platelet count, especially if thrombocytopenia is an isolated, unexpected finding (a clot in the sample bottle is the commonest cause of apparent thrombocytopenia).
3. Bleeding time: Usually prolonged with thrombocytopenia, but unusual prolongation may suggest an additional defect of platelet function (e.g. with leukaemia or myeloproliferative disease).

4. Bone marrow aspiration. Most useful investigation as it will distinguish between failure of production and increased rate of removal from circulation (see above). A biopsy is also useful as it gives a clearer guide to megakaryocyte numbers, but result may not be available for several days. A marrow may also reveal underlying disease such as leukaemia or infiltration.
5. Coagulation screen (see p. 172) to exclude generalised failure of haemostasis (e.g. with DIC).
6. Platelet bound IgG and specific platelet antibodies, if immune thrombocytopenia is suspected. This is only carried out in specialist centres. Arrange with haematology department.

GENERAL MANAGEMENT

In general, thrombocytopenic bleeding associated with failure of platelet production or non-immune causes of increased removal from the circulation can be ameliorated by the transfusion of platelet concentrates.

Platelet infusions in patients with immune thrombocytopenia are usually of no benefit.

For more detailed information see page 207.

DISORDERS OF PLATELET FUNCTION

Usually present with bleeding with a normal or only moderately decreased platelet count but with a very prolonged bleeding time. Platelet count and a bleeding time are the simplest initial investigations, and further laboratory assessment (e.g. in vitro platelet aggregation and measurement of platelet nucleotides) will need to be carried out by specialist laboratories.

Causes

1. Inherited
   e.g. Bernard Soulier syndrome, Glanzman's thrombasthenia, storage pool disease. May need treatment with platelet concentrates to control bleeding.
2. Acquired:
   Commoner
   Drugs e.g. aspirin and other non-steroidal anti-inflammatory agents, penicillins and cephalosporins
   Myeloproliferative diseases
   Renal failure.

REFERENCES

Harker L A, Zimmerman T S (eds) 1983 Platelet disorders. Clinics in Haematology 12(1):
Karpatkin S 1980 Auto-immune thrombocytopenic purpura. Blood 56(3): 329–343
Lilleyman J S 1983 Management of childhood ITP. British Journal of Haematology 54: 11–14
Machin S J 1984 Thrombotic thrombocytopenic purpura. British Journal of Haematology 56:
    191–195

12. LEUCOPENIA

DEFINITION

A total white cell count less than $3.5 \times 10^9/1$. This may result from a decreased neutrophil count, or a decreased neutrophil count *and* lymphocyte count. Agranulocytosis is a term applied to a particularly severe reversible neutropenia usually secondary to drug idiosyncrasy.

Only isolated leucopenia (i.e. normal platelet count and haemoglobin) is considered here. Pancytopenia is dealt with in Chapter 13.

CAUSES

1. Racial variation — particularly in negroes. The neutrophils are largely held in the marginating pool rather than in the circulation.
2. Drugs (see Ch. 35).
3. As a transient phenomenon in viral infections including influenza and other URTIs.
4. Overwhelming pyogenic infection — a combination of peripheral consumption and toxic depression of bone marrow.
5. Myelodysplastic syndromes (Ch. 20).
6. Systemic lupus erythematosus.
7. Familial neutropenia.
8. Cyclical neutropenia.
9. Typhoid fever.
10. Hypersplenism — usually causes pancytopenia, but may cause isolated neutropenia:
    a. Portal hypertension
    b. Tropical splenomegaly
    c. Malignant infiltration of the spleen: leukaemias, lymphomas
    d. Felty's syndrome — rheumatoid arthritis with splenomegaly
    e. Other causes of splenomegaly (see Ch. 16).

POINTS TO NOTE IN HISTORY

1. Drug ingestion.
2. Radiotherapy or cytotoxic chemotherapy.
3. Recent viral infection.
4. Rash or arthritis (SLE).
5. Frequent and severity of recent bacterial infections.
6. Any relatives with similar problems (familial neutropenia).
7. Cyclical nature of symptoms (cyclical neutropenia).
8. History of malarial infection or residence in tropics (tropical splenomegaly).

POINTS TO NOTE ON EXAMINATION

1. Any infected lesions, particularly oral or perineal.
2. Splenomegaly.

INVESTIGATION

1. Blood count and film. Look for neutrophil clumping — a cause of false low WBC counts.
2. ANF and rheumatoid factor.
3. Relevant viral serology and bacterial cultures.
4. Prednisolone stimulation test: give 40 mg of prednisolone after overnight fast and perform neutrophil counts before dose and five hours after. An increment in absolute neutrophil count of more than $2 \times 10^9/1$ indicates that marrow pathology is probably not the cause of the neutropenia. May obviate marrow aspirate, particularly in racial neutropenia.
5. Marrow aspirate — to distinguish peripheral consumption from marrow under-production of leucocytes.
6. Neutrophil antibodies — discuss with laboratory.

Management

1. A neutrophil count of over $1 \times 10^9/1$ is not usually associated with increased susceptibility to infection, and many patients avoid severe infection with neutrophil counts as low as $0.5 \times 10^9/1$.
2. Treat the cause if known e.g. stop drugs.
3. Avoid admission if patient is not infected — hospitals contain resistant pathogenic organisms — but instruct patient to report fever or infective symptoms immediately.

4. Prophylactic antibiotics e.g. half-dose cotrimoxazole 1 tab b.d., and/or anti-thrush agents e.g. amphotericin lozenges sucked q.d.s. may be employed. Consult microbiologist about local policy.
5. If admission to hospital is necessary, use a single room and ban visitors with infections. Local policy may require reverse barrier nursing.
6. Treat any infective episode promptly and vigorously with parenteral antibiotics (see p. 86).

REFERENCES

Dale D C, Guerry D, Wewerka J R, Bull J M, Chusid M J 1979 Chronic neutropenia. Medicine 58(2): 128–136
Logue G L, Shimm D S 1980 Auto-immune granulocytopenia. Annual Review of Medicine 31: 191–200
Minchinton R M, Waters A H 1984 Occurrence and significance of neutrophil antibodies. British Journal of Haematology 56: 521–525

13. PANCYTOPENIA

DEFINITION

Reduction in all the cellular components of the blood — red cells, white cells and platelets.

The above definition simply describes the picture seen in the peripheral blood. It makes no assumptions as to the cause of the abnormality or the functioning of the bone marrow. Pancytopenia may result from:
1. Failure of production.
2. Peripheral destruction.

Some disorders combine both mechanisms.

CAUSES OF PANCYTOPENIA

1. Megaloblastic anaemia. Very common — important because highly treatable (p.16). The anaemia is usually more striking than the leucopenia and thrombocytopenia.
2. Bone marrow infiltration:
   a. Secondary carcinoma
   b. Acute leukaemia (Ch. 18)
   c. Myeloma (Ch. 21)
   d. Myelodysplastic syndromes (Ch. 20)
   e. Myelofibrosis (p. 27)
   f. Lymphoma (Ch. 22)
   g. Osteopetrosis (marble bone disease)
   h. PNH.
3. Splenomegaly with hypersplenism (see Ch. 16).
4. Infection
   a. TB
   b. Overwhelming bacterial sepsis.
5. Aplasia and hypoplasia (p. 79).
6. SLE.

CLINICAL PRESENTATION

Pay particular attention to:
1. Symptoms and signs of bone marrow failure (Ch. 15)

    Anaemia ⎫ Worse in marrow failure than
    Bleeding ⎬ peripheral consumption.
    Infection ⎭

2. Paraesthesiae, atrophic glossitis, family history, previous GIT surgery or small bowel disease (megaloblastic anaemias).
3. Drugs (aplasia).
4. Concurrent infection e.g. TB.
5. Splenomegaly and lymphadenopathy.
6. Symptoms and signs of possible underlying malignancy or connective tissue disorders.

INVESTIGATIONS

Mandatory

1. Blood count with film and differential WBC count, note whether leucoerythroblastic (Ch. 5) due to marrow infiltration, macrocytic (Ch. 6) due to megaloblastic anaemia or primitive WBC due to leukaemia (Ch. 18).
2. Reticulocyte count — may help distinguish between marrow failure and peripheral destruction of RBC.
3. Bone marrow aspirate (+ trephine biopsy if infiltration or aplasia suspected).
4. Serum Vitamin B12, red cell and serum folate levels.
5. Liver function tests.

Most cases will be diagnosable on full clinical examination plus the above simple investigations.

Additional investigations

1. ANF and DNA binding titre, Rheumatoid factor, Ham's test.
2. Screen for TB (cultures, tuberculin test).
3. Other investigations depend on previous clinical and laboratory findings
   e.g. Vitamin B12 absorption tests in megaloblastic anaemia, immunoglobulins in myeloma, lymph node biopsy, lymphangiography or CAT scan in lymphoma.

TREATMENT

Directed to underlying cause. See also chapters on:
1. Aplastic anaemia (Ch. 14).
2. Care of the patient which bone marrow failure (Ch. 15).
3. Blood products (Ch. 29).
4. Splenomegaly (Ch. 16).

14. APLASTIC ANAEMIA

DEFINITION

Pancytopenia (Ch. 13) (often affecting red cells, white cells and platelets to differing extents) due to a hypoplastic marrow, in the absence of marrow fibrosis or malignant cell infiltration. Synonymous with, and perhaps more appropriately known as, hypoplastic anaemia. It is a rare disorder.

The defect in cell production can be at many different stages of haemopoeisis e.g. abnormal marrow microenvironment, decreased numbers of normal stem cells, defective stem cells, changes in humoral or cellular stimulators or inhibitors.

Investigations to establish the nature of the defect are only carried out in research units and the results do not, to date, influence the clinical management.

IMPORTANT FEATURES IN THE HISTORY AND EXAMINATION

1. To establish the cause. (Approximately half of all cases of hypoplastic anaemia remain idiopathic)
   a. Drugs.
      'Expected' myelosuppression — cytotoxic chemotherapy. Dose related or idiosyncratic reaction — almost any drug may be responsible, but the most common are chloramphenicol, chlorpromazine, co-trimoxazole (particularly in the elderly) and non-steroidal anti-inflammatory drugs. Ask about recent travel abroad as chloramphenicol can be bought without a prescription in many countries
   b. Chemicals used at work and with hobbies.
      Particularly solvents (benzene, glues, carbon tetrachloride) and insecticides

   c. Recent viral symptoms (previous three months).
     Particularly linked with hypoplasia are hepatitis A, parvovirus and Epstein-Barr virus. Infectious hepatitis classically causes profound irreversible hypoplasia, unrelated to the clinical severity of the hepatitis
   d. Pregnancy.
     Hypoplasia induced by pregnancy may remit on delivery but is known to recur with subsequent pregnancies
   e. Exposure to ionizing radiation
   f. Look for features of Fanconi's Anaemia (usually presents between the ages of five and ten yers): skeletal anomalies, hypogonadism, skin pigmentation, mental retardation, renal malformations, deafness
   g. History of thrombosis, brown urine — paroxysmal nocturnal haemoglobinuria. Very rare.
2. To establish the clinical severity (see Ch. 15). Hypoplastic anaemia may present with any combination or severity of infection, bleeding and anaemia.

INVESTIGATIONS

1. Blood count with platelet count and leucocyte differential.
2. Blood film: red cells and neutrophils may show dysplastic morphology and macrocytosis.
3. Reticulocyte count. Usually reticulocytes are reduced in number or even absent but paradoxically they may occasionally be normal or even increased (thought to be due to the premature release of reticulocytes from the bone marrow).
4. Bone marrow aspirate (often bloody tap) and trephine biopsy (mandatory to establish the diagnosis). Because of the frequent patchiness of marrow involvement, further trephine biopsies from different sites may be necessary. Send part of the aspirate sample for cytogenetics, helpful in diagnosis of Fanconi's Anaemia and to exclude myelodysplastic syndrome.
5. Viral serology — particularly hepatitis A and Monospot.
6. Pregnancy test.
7. Chest X-rays (AP and lateral) to exclude a thymoma.
8. Ham's acidified test to exclude PNH (contact haematology laboratory).
9. In infants and children, skeletal X-rays (particularly upper limbs) to demonstrate congenital anomalies e.g. absent radii.
10. If available, ^{59}Fe-transferrin isotope studies. Classically show slow plasma iron clearance, reduced utilization and accumulation of isotope in the liver.

11. Neutrophil alkaline phosphatase (NAP) score. This is time-consuming to assess in the presence of severe neutropenia but is a helpful investigation. It is usually high in hypoplastic anaemia.

MANAGEMENT

The treatment and prognosis of hypoplastic anaemia depend on whether it is mild or severe. 'Severe aplastic anaemia' (SAA) is defined by: neutrophil count $< 0.5 \times 10^9/1$, platelets $< 20 \times 10^9/1$, reticulocyte count $< 10 \times 10^9/1$ and bone marrow trephine cellularity of $< 20\%$ haemopoetic cells.

1. Remove any removable cause e.g. drugs, chemicals.
2. All patients under the age of fifty years with SAA are potential candidates for bone marrow transplantation (BMT). As soon as possible after diagnosis, they and their siblings (and parents if young) should be HLA-typed and advice should be sought from the nearest transplant centre re immediate treatment and referral.
3. Observe for two or three weeks to see if spontaneous remission occurs. The severely affected patient will require vigorous supportive treatment during this time (see Ch. 15). Marrow graft survival in SAA after BMT is prejudiced by increasing amounts of pre-transplant blood components, but platelet and blood support must not be withheld from the symptomatic patient. Early referral for transplant is the best way of minimizing exposure to blood components. Never use blood components (e.g. platelets) donated by any member of the family while BMT from a family donor remains a possibility for the patient.
4. If there is no improvement after three weeks, the treatment of choice is:
   a. For patients with SAA and an HLA matched family donor; marrow transplant
   b. For other patients requiring treatment:
      (i) Androgenic steroids: usually given orally e.g. oxymethalone 50 mg t.d.s. Side-effects: cholestatic jaundice, virilism, fluid retention, diarrhoea, growth retardation
      (ii) Corticosteroids in high dose
      (iii) ALG: (anti lymphocyte globulin or anti-thymocyte globulin ATG) raised in rabbits or horses. Given in variable dose as an intravenous infusion in dextrose/saline over four to eight hours. A prior test dose should be given to exclude hypersensitivity to animal protein. Acute anaphylaxis and serum sickness are the principal side-effects.

5. Further treatment depends on the clinical situation e.g.
   a. SAA not responding to ALG and androgens: consider BMT from unrelated donor
   b. Partial response with abnormal blood counts but asymptomatic: observation alone
   c. Persisting anaemia the only problem: consider continuing androgens and maintaining transfusion support.

Prognosis

Very variable. Acute hypoplastic anaemia may be transient or rapidly fatal. Chronic hypoplasia may be unremitting or show transient remissions only. Recovery may be complete or partial — the platelet count is often the last parameter to return to normal and may take several years to do so.

50% of patients with SAA die within three months of diagnosis and 50% of patients with chronic non-severe AA die from the disease within 15 months. The results of BMT are encouraging, particularly with younger patients, but graft failure is still a common problem. New conditioning regimes and improved prophylaxis of graft-versus-host-disease will continue to improve the outlook.

REFERENCES

Comitta B M, Storb R, Thomas E D 1982 Aplastic anaemia: pathogenesis, diagnosis, treatment and prognosis. New England Journal of Medicine 306: 645–652; 712–718
Gale R P, Champlin R E, Feig S A, Fitchen J H 1981 Aplastic anaemia: biology and treatment. Annals of Internal Medicine 95: 477–494
Geary C G 1979 Pathogenesis of aplastic anaemia. British Journal of Hospital Medicine April: 392–402
Thomas E D (ed) 1977 Aplastic anaemia. Clinics in Haematology 7(3):

15. CARE OF THE PATIENT WITH BONE MARROW FAILURE

DEFINITION

Failure of production of normal blood cells.

CAUSES

1. Malignant disease of the bone marrow:
   a. Primary: acute leukaemia (Ch. 18), myeloma (Ch. 21), lymphoma (Ch. 22), myelodysplastic syndromes (Ch. 20)
   b. Secondary: carcinoma.
2. Iatrogenic — induced by chemotherapy or radiotherapy for malignant disease.
3. Aplastic anaemia (Ch. 14).

The most profound pancytopenias are seen during treatment for acute leukaemia, and particularly during bone marrow transplantation. White cell and platelet counts approaching zero are frequently encountered.

Clinical features

1. Anaemia ⎫ The severity of the clinical problem correlates
2. Infection ⎬ well with the degree of depression of peripheral
3. Bleeding ⎭ blood counts.

Severe bone marrow failure may be defined by a neutrophil leucocyte count $< 0.5 \times 10^9/1$, and a platelet count $< 20 \times 10^9/1$.

Prognosis for severe bone marrow failure depends upon its cause and duration. Short periods of pancytopenia are relatively easily tolerated compared with prolonged periods, and infective problems in particular tend to improve quickly if the neutrophil count rises.

MANAGEMENT

General measures

1. Make an assessment of the severity of the problem and its likely outcome. Management of a transplant patient with profound pancytopenia and potentially reversible marrow hypoplasia will differ in intensity from that of a patient with long-standing and resistant disease.
2. Venepuncture and intravenous therapy:
   a. Veins are the patient's lifelines. Venepuncture technique must be aseptic and avoid haematoma formation
   b. Intravenous cannulae should be changed every 24–48 hours
   c. Metal indwelling needles are less traumatic and less liable to infection than polythene cannulae, though may perforate the vein wall if left in for protracted periods
   d. Start with the most peripheral veins for infusions
   e. Skin tunnelled indwelling central venous catheters e.g. Hickman, allow easy access for blood sampling and infusions and are well tolerated by patients (p. 264). Their main drawback is a tendency to introduce infection.
3. Maintaining morale: these patients are very unwell and need expert management. Encouragement and explanation of procedures are very important in keeping up morale. Patients with malignant disease may become significantly depressed and this should be anticipated. Thoughtful use of analgesics, hypnotics and antidepressants may be required.
4. Nutrition: often oral nutrition is difficult because of nausea or oral ulceration. If patients cannot maintain their weight, parenteral nutrition should be considered, including supplements of the B vitamins and vitamin K. Intravenous lipids should be avoided as they may interfere with platelet function.

Correction of anaemia

Use plasma reduced blood to maintain the haemoglobin level at above 10g/dl.

Transfusion reactions may necessitate the use of genotyped, filtered, washed or frozen blood (see Ch. 29). Liaise with the blood bank about this.

Patients with severe thrombocytopenia may undergo a further dilutional drop in the platelet count during transfusion, and therefore when the platelet count is less than $20 \times 10^9/1$, platelet concentrates should be given prior to red cell transfusion wherever possible.

Prevention and treatment of infection

Close liaison with the microbiology department is advantageous. Probability of infection rises steeply as neutrophil count falls.
1. Neutrophils less than $0.5 \times 10^9/1$ — infection probable.
2. Neutrophils less than $0.1 \times 10^9/1$ — infection almost invariable if neutropenia persists.

Main pathogens
Organisms that are ordinarily commensal may cause severe infections in these immunocompromised patients.
1. Bacterial
   a. Gram negative especially E. coli, pseudomonas, klebsiella — often originate from GIT
   b. Staphylococci (often coagulase negative) — often associated with intravenous therapy
   c. Streptococci (often viridans)
   d. Bacteroides (may be mouth or gut derived)
   e. Clostridium (including difficile).
2. Fungal
   Candida is the most common.
3. Viral
   a. Herpes simplex
   b. Cytomegalovirus (associated with immunosuppression rather than neutropenia).

Preventive measures
1. Protective isolation: depends on facilities available e.g.
   a. laminar flow rooms
   b. air filtration
   c. barrier isolation
   d. single room.
   Attendants should be masked and gowned and exhibit scrupulous hand hygiene. Instruments such as stethoscopes should be reserved for individual patients. All routine items of care should preferably be available in the patients room.
   Patients who are neutropenic but well are generally better off at home than in an open ward in hospital.
   If isolation facilities are not available the patient should at least be kept away from patients with active infections.
2. Oral hygiene: the mouth is a common site of ulceration and infection. Antiseptic mouthwashes containing chlorhexidine or povidone-iodine should be used 2–4 hourly. Teeth and gums should be cleaned atraumatically using sponge swabs.

3. Gut decontamination using non absorbable oral antibiotics and anti-fungal agents reduces the population of potentially pathogenic organisms in the intestine.
A suitable regime includes:
   a. Neomycin 500 mg b.d.
   b. Colistin 1.5×10^6 units b.d.
   c. Amphotericin suspension 2 ml q.d.s.
   d. Nystatin suspension 5 ml q.d.s.
4. Avoid routine rectal or vaginal examination because of risk of introducing infection through broken mucous membranes. An intrauterine device should be removed.
5. Food may be sterilised using a suitable microwave cooking process.
Avoid salads, unpeeled fruit and other uncooked foods. Canned foods and drinks are suitable. Utensils should be sterilised.
6. Regular temperature chart (four-hourly).
7. Routine swabs — twice weekly
   a. mouth
   b. nose
   c. perineum
   d. axillae
   e. any skin lesion
   f. cultures of urine, stools, sputum, if appropriate.
8. Prophylactic antibiotics may be useful in the neutropenic patient e.g. co-trimoxazole 1 tab. b.d.; observe local policy.

Treatment of established infection

Febrile episodes (temperature 38°C or more for two hours or 39°C or more for a single reading) should be assumed to be infective in origin unless occurring during transfusion with blood products.

Action

1. Cultures:
   a. blood (including anaerobic and fungal cultures)
   b. urine
   c. sputum if available
   d. swab any lesion
   e. swab drip sites
      (for blood culture sample from both indwelling catheter and peripheral vein).
2. Chest X-ray.
3. Start i.v. antibiotics — suitable combinations are:
Aminoglycoside (e.g. gentamicin, netilmicin, amikacin, tobramycin) *plus* penicillin with broad spectrum and anti-pseudomonal activity (e.g. mezlocillin, ticarcillin, piperacillin) *or* similar cephalosporin.

Common unwanted effects of these combinations include:
a. sodium overload
b. hypokalaemia
c. renal damage
d. ototoxicity.

Careful monitoring of aminoglycoside levels is essential. Use trough and peak samples — consult microbiologist for advice.

Continue antibiotics for forty-eight hours after fever settles and then review subsequent use.

Clinical presentation of infection may determine a variation on routine treatment, e.g. if oral, perineal or gut related add metronidazole to cover anaerobes, if catheter related add extra anti-staphylococcal cover.

Surveillance swabs and cultures during the infective episode may determine treatment changes.

Oral ulceration is commonly due to *Candida* or *Herpes simplex*.

Failure to respond
a. resistant organism
b. fungal or viral infection
c. pneumocystis
d. TB.

May need to start
1. Systemic antifungals: amphotericin (0.25mg/kg once daily as i.v. infusion rising to 1mg/kg if tolerated). Amphotericin may produce fever and is highly nephrotoxic. Pethidine i.v. is useful in preventing rigors and fever. Flucytosine, miconazole and ketoconazole may be useful but are generally inadequate for severe systemic fungal infections.
2. Antiviral therapy: intravenous acyclovir 5mg/kg t.d.s. i.v. infusion for herpetic infection.
3. Granulocyte transfusions (p. 209).

Prevention and treatment of bleeding

1. Careful haemostasis after invasive techniques including venepuncture.
2. No intramuscular injections. Drugs may be given orally, intravenously or subcutaneously.
3. No aspirin-containing products or others likely to interfere with platelet function.
4. Watch for purpura and fundal haemorrhages — use platelet transfusions if present. If platelet count is $< 20 \times 10^9/1$ prophylactic platelet transfusions may be used (p. 207).
5. Exclude other causes of bleeding e.g. DIC, liver disease, renal failure, effect of drugs.

6. Platelet transfusions. 6–12 donor units should be haemostatic in the bleeding patient though only a small increment in platelet count may be produced. Give three times weekly or more frequently if necessary. HLA matched platelets may be available for patients with antibodies (history of reactions or failure to respond to platelet therapy) (p. 208). Consult the blood bank.

7. Tranexamic acid (0.5–1.0g q.d.s. orally or i.v.) may be useful as anti-fibrinolytic therapy to enhance preservation of formed clot. It should not be used with bleeding into the upper urinary tract or closed tissue spaces, or in DIC.

8. Bleeding from specific sites — above measures plus:
   a. Nose bleeds: packing and cautery (often a single troublesome vessel)
   b. GI bleeding:
      (i)   cimetidine/ranitidine
      (ii) usual conservative management
      (iii) avoid operative intervention if at all possible
   c. Vaginal bleeding:
      (i) remote IUCDs
      (ii) progestogen preparation to suppress menstruation.

REFERENCES

Blume K G, Petz L D 1983 In: Zaia J A (ed) Clinical bone marrow transplantation. Churchill Livingstone, Edinburgh, p 131–176
Galea G 1982 Management of bacterial infections in haematological patients. British Journal of Hospital Medicine July: 74–78
Higby D J 1984 In: Goldman J M, Preisler H D (eds) Butterworth, London, p 339–366
Petz L D, Scott E P 1983 In: Zaia J A (ed) Clinical bone marrow transplantation. Churchill Livingstone, Edinburgh, p 177–213

Part 4
ORGANOMEGALY

16. SPLENOMEGALY

A palpably enlarged spleen is usually a reliable sign of disease, though splenomegaly occurs occasionally in apparently normal people. Its causes and investigation depend critically on the normal abode of the patient, as splenomegaly is especially common in the tropics, for a variety of reasons.

HYPERSPLENISM

Defined as an increase in the normal sequestration and destruction of blood cells arising from enlargement of the spleen. It is characterised by:
1. Variable reduction in Hb, WBC count and platelet count.
2. Elevated reticulocyte count.
3. Hypercellular bone marrow.
4. Reversal by splenectomy.
In addition the rise in plasma volume which accompanies splenomegaly may contribute further to the apparent severity of the anaemia.

CAUSES OF SPLENOMEGALY

Primarily haematological

1. Neoplastic:
   a. Leukaemias (chronic lymphocytic including prolymphocytic and hairy-cell leukaemia, chronic granulocytic, acute lymphoblastic and less commonly in acute myeloblastic (Chs 18, 19)
   b. Myelofibrosis (p. 27)
   c. Polycythaemia rubra vera (p. 62)
   d. Myelodysplastic syndromes (Ch. 20)
   e. Lymphoma (Ch. 22)
   f. Histiocytosis X.
2. Non-neoplastic:
   a. Haemolytic anaemias (Ch. 6)
   b. Megaloblastic and iron deficiency anaemias (mild enlargement only)
   c. Autoimmune thrombocytopenia (rare).

91

Non-haematological

1. Infection:
   a. Acute and sub-acute — infectious mononucleosis, endocarditis (bacterial and other), severe pyogenic infection
   b. Chronic — TB, brucellosis, syphilis
   c. Tropical — malaria, leishmaniasis, trypanosomiasis
   The term 'tropical splenomegaly' is generally reserved for chronic splenic enlargement in patients from malarial areas but its occurrence bears no relationship to the apparent severity of infection.
2. Congestive:
   a. Hepatic cirrhosis
   b. Idiopathic portal or splenic vein occlusion.
3. Infiltrative:
   a. Amyloidosis
   b. Mucopolysaccharidoses
   c. Lipid storage disease.
4. Connective tissue disorders:
   a. Rheumatoid arthritis (Felty's syndrome)
   b. Systemic lupus erythematosus.
5. Miscellaneous:
   a. Sarcoidosis
   b. Cysts and haemorrhage
   c. Metastatic tumour
   d. Primary hamartoma

NB: Most likely causes of massive splenomegaly (below umbilicus) in adult patients resident in United Kingdom:

1. Myelofibrosis.
2. Chronic granulocytic leukaemia.
3. Chronic lymphocytic leukaemias.
4. Non-Hodgkin's lymphomas.

POINTS TO NOTE IN HISTORY

1. Pain in splenic area or shoulder tip.
2. Alcohol consumption — portal hypertension secondary to cirrhosis.
3. Recent infections including malaria.
4. Fever or rigors — (SBE).
5. Trauma — splenic haematoma.
6. Previous rheumatic fever (SBE).
7. Neonatal umbilical sepsis (portal vein thrombosis).
8. Abnormal bleeding or bruising — haematological malignancy.
9. Race (congenital haemolytic disorders), e.g. thalassaemia major.
10. Residence and travel abroad.

POINTS TO NOTE ON EXAMINATION

1. Size of spleen (measure in centimetres below costal margin), consistency, tenderness, audible rub.
2. Hepatomegaly.
3. Lymphadenopathy.
4. Fever.
5. Bruising.
6. Oral and other superficial sepsis.
7. Stigmata of liver disease.
8. Stigmata of rheumatoid/SLE.
9. Splinter haemorrhages/fundal haemorrhages.
10. Cardiac murmurs.

INVESTIGATIONS

1. Blood count including red cell indices, reticulocyte count, platelets, differential WBC count, film report (may reveal evidence of haematological malignancy, haemolytic disorders, hypersplenism, eosinophilia in tropical infections).
2. Liver function tests.

   These investigations frequently suggest the diagnosis. If not, then some of the following may be necessary:
3. Bone marrow (±trephine biopsy) — looking for malignant infiltration, megaloblastosis, evidence of hypersplenism, inclusion bodies (e.g. leishmaniasis), storage cells (e.g. Gaucher's disease).
4. Screening tests for haemolysis (Ch. 6) if history or blood count suggestive.
5. Microbiology: blood cultures (if SBE suspected), tuberculin test, cultures for tubercle bacilli, stools for ova, cysts and parasites.
6. Radiology:
   a. Chest (TB, sarcoid, lymphoma)
   b. Abdomen (size of spleen, calcification)
   c. Barium swallow and meal (varices, displacement of organs)
   d. Ultrasound (liver, spleen, portal vein)
   e. CAT scan (liver, spleen, nodes, filling defects, haematomas and cysts)
   f. Radio-isotope scans ($^{99}Tc^m$ colloid or heat damaged ^{51}Cr tagged red blood cells)
   g. Angiography (coeliac axis if abnormal vasculature suspected).
7. Liver biopsy.
8. Laparotomy and splenectomy — ultimate diagnostic tool.

9. Isotopic evaluation of hypersplenism:
Red cell mass, spleen pooling, red cell survival may be measured with ^{51}Cr red cells. Surface counting may give useful information on splenic destruction.

TREATMENT OF SPLENOMEGALY

1. Treat the underlying cause.
2. Splenectomy:
   a. Relative indications: hypersplenism, painful enlargement, haemolysis, or, occasionally, to establish a diagnosis
   b. Avoid if possible in children, especially under the age of five years, because of the increased risk of overwhelming post splenectomy infection with Gram positive organisms
   c. Give oral prophylactic penicillin V (or erythromycin) to all splenectomized children until adulthood. The indications for penicillin prophylaxis in adults is controversial
   d. Give pneumococcal vaccine.

REFERENCES

Bowdler A J 1983 Splenomegaly and hypersplenism. Clinics in Haematology 12(2): 467–488
Richmond J 1980 Hypersplenism. British Journal of Hospital Medicine November: 405–412

17. LYMPHADENOPATHY

Enlarged lymph nodes are often pathological, but must be considered within the context of the patient's age and life style. Children, for instance, usually have large tonsils which would be abnormal in an adult, and people who suffer repeated trauma to the hands and feet often have palpable nodes in the draining areas. Good clinical judgement must determine which nodes require further investigation. Generalised lymphadenopathy may be associated with splenomegaly (Ch. 16).

CAUSES OF LYMPHADENOPATHY

1. Infection
   a. Direct invasion of node by organism, e.g. pyogenic abcess, TB, histoplasmosis, pasteurella
   b. Inflammatory response in regional nodes, draining an infected area, e.g. pyogenic infections, mouth infections, syphilis, and cat scratch fever
   c. Generalised lymphadenopathy, e.g. infectious mononucleosis, toxoplasmosis, syphilis, Rare causes include measles, hepatitis and bacterial endocarditis.
2. Malignancy
   a. Primary lymphoid; lymphoma (Hodgkin's and non-Hodgkin's, Ch. 22). Leukaemia (chronic lymphocytic, acute lymphoblastic (Chs 18, 19)
   b. Secondary invasion; carcinoma, myeloid leukaemias.
3. Immune
   a. SLE
   b. Rheumatoid
   c. Drug reactions
   d. Serum sickness.
4. Miscellaneous
   a. Sarcoidosis
   b. Hyperthyroidism
   c. AIDS
   d. Histiocytic medullary reticulosis
   e. In association with chronic skin diseases.

Localised lymphadenopathy is most likely to be due to local infection, secondary tumour or early stage lymphoma.

POINTS OF PARTICULAR NOTE IN HISTORY

1. Age, occupation, sexual orientation (AIDS).
2. Fever, weight loss, sweats (lymphoma, infections).
3. Local discomfort (pyogenic infection).
4. Local infection or trauma.
5. Pruritus (lymphoma, skin diseases).
6. Joint pains (rheumatoid, SLE).
7. Drugs.
8. Other symptoms suggestive of an underlying disorder.

POINTS OF PARTICULAR NOTE ON EXAMINATION

Nodes

1. Size.
2. Consistency
   a. Fluctuant in abscess formation
   b. Hard in carcinoma, TB
   c. Rubbery in lymphoma.
3. Mobility and attachment to skin or subcutaneous tissues.
4. Superficial inflammation or ulceration.
5. Sinus formation.
6. Tenderness.
7. Distribution.

Other organs

1. Spleen and liver, size and consistency.
2. Infectious lesions in area draining to nodes.
3. Joint swelling.
4. Other signs of systemic disease.
5. Examination of post nasal space in unexplained localised cervical lymphadenopathy.
6. Skin disease.

INVESTIGATIONS

1. Nodes considered definitely pathological:
   a. FBC — look for evidence of haematological malignancy, viral or other infection
      Bone marrow at this stage if FBC suggests haematological malignancy
   b. Glandular fever screening test
   c. Serology for toxoplasma and syphilis
   d. Microbiological — culture possible infected lesions or areas draining to nodes, e.g. throat swab
   e. Tuberculin test
   f. Chest X-ray (TB, lymphoma, sarcoidosis)
   g. Aspiration cytology (especially if metastatic carcinoma suspected). If unsuccessful:
   h. Lymph node biopsy (avoid inguinal nodes if possible — cervical nodes ideal)
      (i)   'imprint' from cut surface of node
      (ii) immunological studies on fresh tissue
            (not in formalin if lymphoma suspected — liaise with laboratory).
      (iii) culture including TB.
   Other investigations will depend on result of biopsy, and evidence clinically of systemic disease, e.g. rheumatoid factor, anti-HTLV III antibodies if AIDS suspected etc.
2. Nodes of uncertain significance:
   a. Perform non-invasive investigations from list above
   b. Observe progression of nodes over short period of few weeks at most
   c. If not definitely resolved biopsy after period of observation.
3. Nodes with unresolved histology: patients having nodes with non-diagnostic granulomatous changes or reactive hyperplasia should be observed and re-biopsied if diagnosis still uncertain, after a reasonable interval. Subsequent biopsy may show progression to lymphoma.

TREATMENT

This is related entirely to cause.

REFERENCE

Zuelzer W W, Kaplan J 1975 The child with lymphadenopathy. Seminars in Haematology 12(3): 323–333

Part 5
MALIGNANT
HAEMATOLOGICAL
DISEASE

18. ACUTE LEUKAEMIA (AL)

DEFINITION

A primary malignancy of haemopoietic cells characterized by replacement of normal bone marrow by primitive blast cells, and the appearance of such cells in the peripheral blood. Usually rapidly progressive and fatal without treatment.

CLASSIFICATION

Classification depends upon identification of recognisable (though abnormal) features of a particular cell line.

Acute myeloid leukaemia (AML)

The FAB (French/American/British) classification recognises six types (M1 — M6) based on bone marrow morphology:

    M1 — acute myeloblastic (undifferentiated)
    M2 — acute myeloblastic (with some degree of differentiation)
    M3 — promyelocytic
    M4 — myelomonocytic
    M5 — pure monocytic
    M6 — acute erythroleukaemia.

Clinical presentation may vary between types but no *definite* difference prognostically has been identified as yet between these groups. Clinical trials may yet elucidate this.

Acute undifferentiated leukaemia
Cells have pleomorphic appearance but no classifiable features.

Acute megakaryoblastic leukaemia
Recently recognised clinical entity characterised by atypical small megakaryocytes or small densely basophilic blasts. Often causes secondary marrow fibrosis.

Acute lymphoblastic leukaemia (ALL)

Usually classified *immunologically* on the basis of surface marker studies:
Common ALL (possessing the common ALL antigen: c-ALL)
T cell type (T-ALL)
B cell type (B-ALL or Burkitt's type)
Null (non B, non T and lacking cALL antigen).
These sub-divisions have differing clinical presentations, response to treatment and ultimate prognosis (c-ALL has best long term prognosis and B-ALL the worst).
May also be classified *morphologically* (by FAB):
L1 — small blasts with scanty cytoplasm
L2 — larger, more pleomorphic, more cytoplasm, more obvious nucleoli
L3 — densely basophilic, vacuolated cytoplasm.
L1 and L2 may have cALL or T-ALL or null phenotypes but within each group L1 has a better prognosis. L3 corresponds to B-ALL and has universally poor outlook.

Acute transformation of chronic granulocytic leukaemia
(see also Ch. 19)

Commonly CGL transforms into an acute phase behaving as a poor prognosis acute leukaemia. Most commonly AML but ALL, undifferentiated, mixed and megakaryoblastic all described. Characteristically the blasts retain the Philadelphia chromosome (Ph^1 — translocation from long arm of chromosome 22 to long arm of chromosome 9), plus further chromosome abnormalities. Full classification of AL takes into account:

1 *Clinical features* (q.v.).
2. *Morphology of blood* and bone marrow, including specific *cytochemical stains* e.g. PAS, peroxidase, Sudan black, non-specific esterase, acid phosphatase.
3. *Immunological markers* on blast cells, including typing using monoclonal antisera.
4. *Specific cellular enzymes* e.g. TdT (terminal deoxynucleotidyl transferase), lyzozyme, lactoferrin.
5. *Chromosome studies* on bone marrow. Some have characteristic translocations. Minor anomalies are being increasingly identified by modern culture and banding techniques, especially in AML.
6. *Cell culture patterns* — especially AML — may be of prognositic significance.
See Table 18.1.

Table 18.1 Classification of acute leukaemia

Main group	Sub type	Prominent clinical features	Morphological (FAB) classification	Diagnostic tests
Acute lymphoblastic	Common ALL (cALL)		L1 or L2	cALL antigen +ve, TdT +ve PAS +ve blocks in cytoplasm
	T-ALL	Thymic enlargement	L1 or L2	TdT +ve, anti-T + ve Acid phosphatase +ve
	B-ALL	Spleen Liver Nodes	L3	Surface immunoglobulin +ve 14, 8 chromosomal translocation
Acute myeloid	Myeloblastic		M1 or M2	Sudan Black +ve. Auer rods ±
	Promyelocytic	DIC	M3	Sudan Black + Auer rods common Granules common. 15, 17 translocation
	Myelomonocytic	Gum hyperplasia	M4	Non-specific esterase +ve
	Monoblastic	Gum hyperplasia Nodes, Liver Spleen	M5	Sudan Black +ve Non-specific esterase +ve
Megakaryoblastic	Erythroleukaemia		M6	PAS +ve erythroblasts Platelet peroxidase +ve PAS +ve. Bone marrow fibrosis common

AETIOLOGY OF ACUTE LEUKAEMIA

Known predisposing factors:
1. Radiation — effects of large doses clearcut but smaller 'background' doses have uncertain role.
2. Chemicals — e.g. benzene.
3. Cytotoxic drugs — AL increasingly seen in patients successfully treated for other malignancies. Combinations of radiotherapy and chemotherapy seem to be particularly risky.
4. Viruses and oncogenes.

CLINICAL FEATURES

1. Usually short history.
2. Bone marrow failure (see also Ch. 15)
   a. *Anaemia*, often severe
   b. *Bleeding*: skin — bruising, purpura
                    gums
                    nose
                    GI tract
                    GU tract
                    CNS haemorrhage
   c. *Infection*: mouth — oral ulceration in association with Candida, Herpes simplex or bacterial infection
                    perineum
                    skin lesions
                    lung
                    oesophageal Candidiasis.
3. Tissue infiltration
   a. Lymphadenopathy, splenomegaly — especially in ALL, (more so in T and B-ALL) and M5 AML
   b. Bone pain, joint swelling
   c. Gum hyperplasia (monocytic)
   d. CNS disease (especially ALL)
   e. Testicular swelling (especially ALL)
   f. Renal failure
   g. Lung infiltration
   h. Skin lesions ('leukaemids')
   i. Thymic enlargement (T-ALL, may cause respiratory difficulties or simply anterior mediastinal mass on chest X-ray).
4. General symptoms — weight loss, fever, sweating, malaise, anorexia.
5. Others:
   a. Hyperuricaemia leading to gout and renal failure
   b. Disseminated intravascular coagulation (especially promyelocytic).

POINTS TO NOTE IN HISTORY

1. Recent infections.
2. Sibling details (may be relevant if bone marrow transplant a possibility or for HLA matched blood products).
3. Presence of intra-uterine device — possible source of infection and bleeding, should be removed.

POINTS TO NOTE ON EXAMINATION

1. Pyrexia — always assume this is infective in origin.
2. Purpura — especially fundal: presence indicates severe thrombocytopenia and danger of serious (e.g. CNS) haemorrhage.
3. Oral ulceration.
4. CNS abnormalities, especially papilloedema and cranial nerve lesions.
5. Infective lesions, especially around perineum, as these are often very serious.
6. Signs of systemic infection, especially chest.
7. Do not perform vaginal or rectal examination unless good clinical indication as this is liable to introduce infection.
8. Signs of leucostasis. Hyperviscosity from very high WBC count (confusion, lung infiltrates, venous congestion in fundi, papilloedema).
9. Avoid too frequent BP readings unless clinically indicated as this may cause purpura on arms.

INVESTIGATIONS TO ESTABLISH DIAGNOSIS

1. FBC with film, differential WBC count, platelets. May be nucleated RBC, myelocytes, as well as blasts. May simply be pancytopenic without blasts (aleukaemic leukaemia) — commoner in ALL.
2. Bone marrow aspirate for:
   a. Routine morphology and cytochemistry.
3. Where indicated/available:
   a. Chromosome studies (especially AML and CGL in transformation)
   b. Immunological markers (e.g. cALL Antigen, T and B markers, Ia marker)
   c. Enzyme assays (e.g. TdT in ALL; lyzozyme in AML)
   d. In vitro culture.
4. Bone marrow trephine may give additional information on degree of infiltration. May show secondary fibrosis.
5. Serum lyzozome level (AML especially monocytic).

OTHER INVESTIGATIONS

Once diagnosis established various baseline investigations relevant to future management should be initiated.

Haematological
1. Blood group and antibody screen.
2. HLA type (necessary for transplantation, blood products; often not possible until remission because of low lymphocyte count).
3. Coagulation screen to exclude DIC.

Biochemical
1. Renal function screen.
2. Urate.
3. Liver function screen.
4. Serum calcium (magnesium if available).

Microbiological
1. Superficial surveillance swabs — include mouth, skin, nose, perineum.
2. Urine and stool culture.
3. Blood cultures (and any other clinically indicated) if febrile.
4. Baseline viral titres (especially HSV and CMV).
5. Hepatitis surface antigen.

Radiological
1. Chest X-ray
2. Others where clinically indicated.

MANAGEMENT

Falls into two main categories:
1. Supportive treatment.
2. Definitive anti-leukaemic treatment.

Supportive treatment

See Ch. 15 for care of the patient with bone marrow failure, with special reference to prevention and treatment of infection, and bleeding. *Blood products* are discussed in Ch. 29.
1. Maintain Hb > 10g/dl by transfusion of packed cells.
2. Platelet transfusions (p 207) are indicated when:
   a. There is clinical evidence of bleeding e.g. purpura
   b. When transfusion with stored blood may dilute an already low platelet count
   c. Prophylactic platelet transfusions are often used when the count falls below $20 \times 10^9/1$. Such use depends on local availability and policy.

3. Prevent urate nephropathy and gout due to rapid cell lysis:
   a. Start allopurinol 300 daily (or b.d. with high tumour load) preferably at least 24 hours before chemotherapy
   b. Ensure good fluid input and output with careful records of balance.
4. Check electrolytes daily or more frequently during initial stages of treatment — cell lysis may cause hyperkalaemia.
5. Combinations of chemotherapy, antibiotics and infection lead to other metabolic problems. Keep a check on:
   a. Renal and liver function
   b. K^+, Ca^{++}, Mg^{++} levels
   c. Albumin (may reflect poor nutrition) (p. 84).
6. Coagulation screen (PT, APPT, TT): liver infiltration, certain drugs e.g. asparaginase may cause coagulation defects. DIC is common in promyelocytic leukaemia and may occur in any AL especially after cell lysis. Heparin in low dose may be useful but must be very carefully monitored (see Ch. 27).
7. Arrange insertion of Hickman catheter if possible (see Ch. 38).
8. Maintain the patient's morale. Careful discussion and explanation of disease and treatment are extremely important. Be honest and optimistic as far as reasonably possible. Use anti-emetics, analgesia and psychotropic drugs where indicated. Consider sedation/anaesthesiae for painful procedures in children and nervous adults.

Definitive chemotherapy

This aims at elimination of the leukaemic cell population with regeneration of normal marrow. Cure or long term survival is the goal.

Remission is defined as:
   1. No excess of blasts in bone marrow.
   2. Normal peripheral blood counts.

Stages of treatment:
   1. Remission induction.
   2. Remission consolidation.
   3. Maintenance of remission.

Duration of first remission correlates closely with survival and in general patients who relapse will die soon of their disease. In general the more intensive the induction and consolidation regimes the more likely a remission is to be achieved and maintained. Most modern regimes are based on this premise. Patients should be treated for AL only in centres which have experienced and expert staff.

AML

Induction chemotherapy
Initial treatment usually includes the following:

      1. i.v. anthracycline e.g. daunorubicin, Adriamycin
                            +

      2. i.v./s.c. cytosine arabinoside
                            +

      3. Oral 6-thioguanine

Second line drugs include:
M-AMSA
Etoposide
Mitoxantrone

The regimes are highly myelotoxic and in order to achieve a remission a period of bone marrow aplasia is inevitable.

Remission induction may be achieved after a single course or may require several, depending on intensity of courses and disease response.

Consolidation utilises similar drug regimes once remission achieved.

Remission maintenance
In young patients with a histocompatible sibling, bone marrow transplantation after total body irradiation may offer the best chance of long term survival.

Regular chemotherapy for maintenance usually utilises the same drugs as induction, without the anthracycline and in lower dosage. Efficacy of maintenance treatment in AML is doubtful.

ALL

Remissions are more readily achieved than in AML and prolonged aplasia need not necessarily occur. There is good evidence however that remission duration is prolonged after intensive induction and consolidation, especially in poor prognostic groups, and so the most recent regimes have adopted this approach. During this phase the patient may therefore be rendered severely pancytopenic.

Induction consolidation chemotherapy
Combinations of:
    vincristine
        +
    adriamycin/daunorubicin
        +
    prednisolone
        +
    cytosine arabinoside
        +
    methotrexate (medium to high dose)
        +
    l-asparaginase

In addition CNS prophylaxis is given in the form of intrathecal methotrexate ± cytosine arabinoside ± cranial irradiation.

Remission maintenance
Of established importance in ALL. May be continuous or interrupted and mainly consists of oral medication.

Drugs used in maintenance: methotrexate
6 mercaptopurine
prednisolone
cytosine arabinoside
(occasional vincristine, anthracycline)

Complications
1. Relapse in bone marrow. Almost always means disease incurable by conventional techniques. Further remission induction may be possible using original or different drugs. If achieved consider bone marrow transplant in ALL if suitable patient and donor.
2. CNS disease. May be present at diagnosis or develop after bone marrow remission. Clinical presentation — usually as leukaemic meningitis — headaches, papilloedema, cranial nerve palsies, vomiting. More common in ALL, hence prophylactic therapy. Increasingly seen in AML as more prolonged remissions achieved and prophylaxis in AML is now more widely used. If develops despite prophylaxis the same drugs are used and irradiation may be repeated once.

Cranial irradiation
18–24 Gy over two and a half to three weeks.
Complications:
a. Leuco-encephalopathy — unusual but serious, usually fatal — also seen with i.t. methotrexate.
b. 'Somnolent syndrome' — seen six to ten weeks after irradiation, commonly benign course.
c. Mild intellectual (especially mathematical) impairment in children.
3. Testicular disease. Seen in 10% of male ALL. Presents with painless often bilateral swelling. May herald CNS or bone marrow relapse. Treatment:
a. Irradiation (sometimes done prophylactically)
b. Further systemic ± CNS therapy.
4. Immunosuppression. Especially seen in ALL.
Viral infections such as measles, chickenpox may be fatal. Give i.m. gamma globulin (hyperimmune for chickenpox/zoster) if patient exposed. School children especially susceptible. Keep away from school if cases occur in class and give gamma globulin.

Do not give BCG or routine vaccinations involving live viruses; avoid rubella, measles, oral polio, smallpox and yellow fever and some influenza vaccines.
5. Infertility. Very likely especially in males. Inevitable after radiotherapy to gonads. Some females and occasional males fertile and have normal offspring. Sperm storage should be considered before chemoradiotherapy started.

PROGNOSIS

AML

> 70% obtain first remission in most series with present day regimes. Remission duration and survival vary between series, some put four year remission duration as high as 20%.

Poor prognostic features:
1. Very high WBC count on presentation especially if $> 100 \times 10^9/1$. Survival very poor.
2. Preceeding pre-leukaemic phase (see Ch. 20).
3. Cell type and karyotype may have prognostic implications.
4. Increasing age.

ALL

Remission obtained: > 95% in cALL
　　　　　　　　　　lower in T-ALL
　　　　　　　　　　much lower in B-ALL
Overall six year survival in children 50%
(i.e. long term cure probable).
Much less in adults.
Poor prognostic features:
1. High WBC on presentation i.e. $> 20 \times 10^9/1$
   If $> 100 \times 10^9/1$ very few survive one year.
2. Age if < 2 or > 10 years.
3. T cell or especially B cell disease.
4. Males.
5. Abnormal karyotype.
6. L3 or L2 morphology.
7. CNS disease on presentation.

REFERENCES

Bloomfield C D 1984 Acute lymphoblastic leukaemia. In: Goldman J M, Preisler H D (eds) Leukaemias. Butterworth, London, p 163–189
Boros L, Bennett J M The acute myeloid leukaemias. In: Goldman J M, Preisler H D (eds) Leukaemias. Butterworth, London p 104–135
Foon K A, Schroff R W, Gale R P 1982 Surface markers on leukaemia and lymphoma cells: recent advances. Blood 60(1): 1–19
Lister T A, Rohatiner A Z S The management of acute myeloid leukaemia. In: Goldman J M, Preisler H D (eds) Leukaemias. Butterworth, London, p 136–162

19. CHRONIC LEUKAEMIAS

DEFINITION

Primary malignancies of haemopoietic cells in which the clinical course is measured in months and years in contrast to the acute leukaemias.

Many of the malignant cells are differentiated and these relatively mature cells appear in large numbers in the peripheral blood, giving rise to a leucocytosis which may be very marked.

CLASSIFICATION

Myeloid origin

1. Chronic granulocytic (synonymous myeloid) — CGL or CML.
2. Chronic myelomonocytic (CMML).
3. Chronic erythroleukaemia (Di Guglielmo's syndrome).

Lymphoid origin

1. Chronic lymphocytic (B-cell or T-cell).
2. Prolymphocytic (B-cell or T-cell).
3. Hairy cell (leukaemic reticuloendotheliosis).

CHRONIC MYELOID (GRANULOCYTIC) LEUKAEMIA

Malignant clone derives from a committed stem cell, and differentiates along myeloid lines. In 95% of cases the Philadelphia chromosome (Ph[1]), a number 22 chromosome missing part of its long arm which has become attached to chromosome 9 (t (22;9)), is present in the affected clone in bone marrow and blood. Myeloid, erythroid, megakaryocytic and some lymphoid cells carry the Ph[1] chromosome.

Clinical presentation

1. Typically middle age, but seen in all age groups.
2. Enlarged spleen and liver (splenomegaly may be massive and cause discomfort).
3. May present asymptomatically on routine blood count.
4. Symptoms of anaemia.
5. Abnormal bleeding.
6. Weight loss, anorexia, sweats, fever, 2° amenorrhoea.
7. Hyperviscosity syndrome from leucostasis.
8. Gout.
9. De novo 'blast transformation' clinically indistinguishable from acute leukaemia.

Severe infection is rare in untreated CGL (unlike all other types of leukaemia) as the relatively mature myeloid cells seen in the blood have some bacteriocidal capabilities.

Clinical signs

1. Splenomegaly: may vary from just palpable to massive and may have audible rub or bruit.
2. Hepatomegaly.
3. Pallor, emaciation (if advanced).
4. Bruising (seldom petechial, except in blast transformation).
5. Fever (low grade, even in absence of infection).
6. Fundal haemorrhages, tortuous veins, papilloedema (leucostasis).
7. Bone tenderness, especially sternum.
8. Lymphadenopathy (rare).
9. Skin infiltration (uncommon).

Investigations

Blood count

1. Leucocytosis may be very marked, often well over $100 \times 10^9/1$. Height of leucocytosis tends to correlate with size of spleen and degree of anaemia.
2. Differential leucocyte count: whole spectrum from neutrophils (around 50%) to blasts (usually < 5%). Myelocytes common. Eosinophils and basophils increased.
   Nucleated RBCs often seen.
3. Anaemia: normochromic, normocytic, may be mild or severe.
4. Thrombocytosis sometimes $> 1000 \times 10^9/1$. Platelets occasionally low — may herald blast transformation.

The diagnosis is often obvious from the clinical signs and the blood count alone, in classical CGL.

Bone marrow

1. Grossly hypercellular.
2. May be difficult to aspirate.
3. Gross granulocytic hyperplasia with all degrees of differentiation seen, and increased megakaryocytes.
4. Send sample for examination for Ph^1 and other chromosome anomalies (liaise with laboratory about sample — marrow or blood anticoagulated with heparin is suitable).
5. Marrow trephine to assess fibrosis; may also show pockets of blasts not detected on aspirate, in early transformation.

Note: If Ph^1 chromosome detected in peripheral blood cells it may not always be necessary to perform a bone marrow.

Additional investigations (once diagnosis made or suspected).

1. Urate — often very high.
2. NAP score — neutrophil alkaline phosphatase zero or very low in untreated CML, in contrast to other causes of leucocytosis. Tends to rise after control of WBC, or before blast transformation.
3. Liver function — deranged enzymes and mildly raised bilirubin common.
4. Renal function — as baseline.
5. Serum vitamin B12 level and binding proteins if available. (Transcobalamin secreted by leucocytes is raised in CML and other myeloproliferative diseases, giving rise to high serum vitamin B12 level.)

Management

1. Aim generally is to control the clinical and haematological manifestations of the disease. True remission is seldom achieved in that the Ph^1 chromosome is almost always still detectable in bone marrow. Newer more radical approaches to treatment may prove to be useful in prolonging survival.
2. Start Allopurinol as soon as possible.
3. Leucapheresis. This involves harvesting leucocytes from peripheral blood by means of a cell separator. Two main purposes:
   a. Rapid, safe reduction in WBC count where leucostasis is giving rise to clinical problems
   b. Storage of peripheral blood cells for future autograft if this becomes necessary. Such harvests contain large numbers of stem cells capable of marrow engraftment. (In addition to harvested cells may be useful in providing leucocyte support to severely neutropenic patients and are safe for this provided they are irradiated first.)

4. Chemotherapy. Aim at reducing WBC count to a level at which the patient is asymptomatic e.g. 5-25 × 10^9/1. Achieving this will also usually control the anaemia, thrombocytosis, and splenomegaly, though occasionally these remain as specific problems. Symptoms will also improve as the counts become normal. When count well controlled often the only sign of disease is persistent eosinophilia and basophilia and reduced NAP score. Occasional myelocytes may remain.

Drugs used include:

a. Hydroxyurea: usually 0.5–2.0 g daily. Well tolerated, good control of counts without long term marrow or other toxicity. Effect short lived so has to be given daily or alternate days as a rule.

b. Busulphan: 2–4 mg daily. May also be given as single large dose intermittently e.g. 1 mg/kg monthly. Intermittent dosage may result in less long term toxicity. Well tolerated generally. Inadvertent overdosage may cause fatal aplasia. Causes amenorrhoea in females and hypofertility in males. Long term problems include pulmonary fibrosis, mutagenicity.

c. 6-Mercaptopurine. 50–150 mg daily. Reduce dose if concurrent allopurinol administration.

d. 6-Thioguanine. 40–160 mg daily.

Combinations sometimes useful if control difficult e.g. busulphan + thioguanine. More intensive treatment regimes similar to those used in AML have been tried in an attempt to improve prognosis, so far without conspicuous success.

5. Splenectomy. Has been advocated as a means of removing a potential source of blast transformation. May make palliative management of blast crises easier but does not avert this or improve prognosis. May also cause intractable thrombocytosis. Not generally advocated.

6. Supportive treatment. Transfusion may be necessary in early stages but should be avoided when WBC very high as may aggravate hyperviscosity. Hb levels of 8–9 g/dl are well tolerated and will improve as WBC controlled. Regular transfusion may become necessary in later stages.

7. Bone marrow transplant. May have a place if histocompatible donor available and patient young (perhaps < 40 years). Long term results unknown.

Disease progression

At present time CML is incurable by conventional techniques. Median survival is approximately three years. After the initial chronic phase disease in which the patient is clinically well, one of two main terminal states develop:

1. *Blast transformation*: a more malignant clone appears which gives rise to progeny which are primitive blast cells. The result is a slow or abrupt transformation to an acute leukaemia, of particularly resistant type, with appearance of increased numbers of blasts in marrow and peripheral blood.

   Blasts often have additional chromosome anomalies as well as Ph[1]. May be of any phenotype: i.e. AML, ALL, undifferentiated or megakaryoblastic. Some CML patients present for first time in this phase.

   Treatment is that of acute leukaemia. Remission rates and duration less than straightforward AL, and patients who respond revert back to chronic phase disease. Grafting with autologous buffy coat cells (obtained at diagnosis by leucapheresis and cryopreserved), after intensive chemotherapy or radiotherapy, has been used, but long term results poor.

2. *Bone marrow failure*. Some patients do not enter a discernible blast crisis but develop insidious marrow failure with progressive anaemia, thrombocytopenia and splenomegaly. Marrow often very fibrotic. May be natural disease process or related to chemotherapy, particularly busulphan. Patients often emaciated and hypercatabolic. Treatment is supportive only.

JUVENILE CHRONIC MYELOID LEUKAEMIA

Adult-type CGL does occur occasionally in childhood, usually in older age group. Juvenile chronic myeloid leukaemia is a distinct rare disease.

Clinical features

1. Age < 2 years.
2. Mild splenomegaly.
3. Lymphadenopathy.
4. Facial rash.

Laboratory features

1. Thrombocytopenia.
2. Increased monocytes and blasts in blood and marrow.
3. Many nucleated RBC.
4. High Hb F level.
5. Absence of Ph^1 chromosome.

Treatment

Response to treatment is poor. Approximate survival < one year.

CHRONIC MYELOMONOCYTIC LEUKAEMIA

May be classified either as a type of myelogenous leukaemia or as a myelodysplastic syndrome (see Ch. 20).

Clinical and laboratory features

1. Elderly patient.
2. Chronic course often over several years.
3. Leucocytosis with absolute increase in monocytes and some abnormal forms in blood and bone marrow.
4. Splenomegaly.
5. Anaemia and thrombocytopenia.

Treatment

1. Treatment is generally supportive, and many patients do relatively well.
2. Gentle chemotherapy e.g. 6-mercaptopurine or hydroxyurea may be useful in controlling very high WBC count and splenomegaly, and may improve anaemia and thrombocytopenia.

CHRONIC ERYTHROLEUKAEMIA (syn. Di Guglielmo's syndrome, chronic erythraemic myelosis)

A chronic variation of which the acute counterpart is M6 AML.

Clinical features

Chronic form usually presents with anaemia and runs a course over months and years. Splenomegaly may be present.

Laboratory features

1. Anaemia.
2. Increased reticulocytes.
3. Numerous nucleated RBC in blood.
4. Gross erythroid hyperplasia in marrow.
5. PAS +ve erythroblasts in marrow.
6. Variable dysmyelopoiesis.
7. May terminate as AML.

Treatment

1. Transfusion.
2. Chemotherapy e.g. 6-MP may be useful in some cases.

CHRONIC LYMPHOID LEUKAEMIAS

Can be classified:

1. Clinically.
2. Morphologically. ⎫
3. Immunologically. ⎭   See Table 19.1.

Generally the malignant clone has a normal counterpart in lymphocyte development, but the cells have aberrant features and are functionally defective.

B-CELL CHRONIC LYMPHOCYTIC LEUKAEMIA (B-CLL)

Commonest form of leukaemia in United Kingdom. Affects mainly elderly — very rare below thirty. Often detected on routine blood count as an absolute lymphocytosis. CLL is the most common cause of persistent lymphocytosis in a middle aged or elderly patient.

Clinical features

1. Often asymptomatic with no abnormal physical signs.
2. Lymphadenopathy — all areas, soft, may be very extensive.
3. Hepatosplenomegaly.
4. Weight loss, night sweats, fatigue, recurrent infections.

Disease progression.

Table 19.1

Disease	Sub-type	Morphology	Immunology
Chronic lymphocytic leukaemia (CLL)	B-cell	Small round lymphocyte	sIg +ve (IgM ± D)
		'Smudge cells'	'Mouse' rosettes +++ve
			Normal equivalent a very early B-lymphocyte
	T-cell (very rare in UK)	More cytoplasm than B-cell	Anti-T +ve
		Acid phosphatase +ve granules	'E' rosettes
			Mostly T suppressor cells
		(HTLV associated has bizarre convoluted appearance)	(Anti HTLV +ve)
Prolymphocytic leukaemia (PLL)	B-cell	Large cell with single nucleolus	sIg +++ve (IgM ± D)
			'Mouse' rosettes ±ve
			Normal equivalent a later B lymphocyte
	T-cell (20% of all PLL)	Same as B-PLL	Anti T +ve
			'E' rosettes ±ve
			Mostly T helper cells
Hairy cell leukaemia (HCL)	B-cell	Characteristic 'hairy' cell	sIg +++ve (IgM + G + A)
		Fibrosis	'Mouse' rosettes +ve
	T-cell	As above	As T-CLL and T-PLL.

Laboratory features

1. Absolute lymphocytosis $> 15 \times 10^9/1$. WBC may be very high 500–600 $\times 10^9/1$.
2. 'Smudge' cells or 'smear' cells (lymphocytes ruptured on spreading film) characteristic.
3. Anaemia, neutropenia and thrombocytopenia develop as the disease progresses.

Staging

Three main staging systems based on clinical and haematological parameters. All assume diagnosis based on minimum criteria of:

1. Peripheral blood lymphocytosis $> 15 \times 10^9/1$.
2. Bone marrow lymphocytosis $> 40\%$.

Simplest classification is as follows:

Stage A: Hb > 10 g/dl. Platelets > 100 x $10^9/1$.
       < 3 lymphoid areas involved.

Stage B: Hb > 10 g/dl. Platelets > 100 x $10^9/1$.
       3 or more lymphoid areas involved.

Stage C: Hb < 10 g/dl, OR Platelets < 100 x $10^9/1$.
       Regardless of lymphoid areas involved.

Worsening prognosis.

NB: 1. A lymphoid area includes liver, or spleen or a single group of nodes e.g. neck, axillae, groins.
2. Level of lymphocyte count not considered prognostically important although counts tend to rise as disease progresses.
3. Anaemia and thrombocytopenia excludes that caused by a definite auto-immune process.

Complications

1. Infections. CLL patients suffer increasing immunosuppression as disease progresses with reduced normal immunoglobulins and defective cell mediated responses. A monoclonal paraprotein may be present.
   Viral infections, especially Herpes zoster and simplex, and bacterial infections, especially pneumonia, are common.
2. Auto-immune phenomena. Positive direct antiglobulin (Coombs) test in 5–10%.
   Antibody may be warm or cold in type. May or may not lead to haemolysis. Immune thrombocytopenia may also occur.
3. Hyperviscosity: if WBC reaches 400–500 × $10^9/1$ or more.
4. Hyperuricaemia.

Investigations

1. Full blood count and reticulocytes, film, direct antiglobulin test.
2. Peripheral blood for lymphocyte markers, "mouse rosettes" and 'sIg' (surface immunoglobulin) if available.
3. Bone marrow aspirate and trephine. A 'nodular' pattern of lymphocyte infiltration on trephine may suggest better prognosis than diffuse infiltrate.
4. Renal and liver function.
5. Uric acid.
6. Protein electrophoresis and immunoglobulin levels.
7. Chest X-ray.

Treatment

1. Not always necessary. Do not treat high white count per se unless causing hyperviscosity.
   Indications for treatment include: severe symptoms such as night sweats, weight loss; anaemia or thrombocytopenia; bulky palpable disease.
2. Patients with high uric acid require allopurinol e.g. 300 mg o.d.
3. First line drugs — chlorambucil ± steroids. Can be given continuously in low dose e.g. 2–6 mg chlorambucil daily, or intermittently e.g. 10–25 mg daily for one week in three, or more. The latter approach may be less immunosuppressive and more effective.
   Prednisolone is especially useful for auto-immune phenomena.
4. For resistant disease COP (cyclophosphamide, vincristine and prednisolone) or even CHOP (cyclophosphamide, adriamycin, vincristine, and prednisolone) may be useful. Details of these drugs are given in Ch. 23.
5. Radiotherapy. Low dose to bulk disease often useful. Total body irradiation in small weekly doses to a total of 100–200 rads is well tolerated and an alternative to chemotherapy.
   Splenic irradiation may also be useful.
6. Supportive treatment. Blood transfusion — may need to initiate a regular regime for progressive anaemia. Prompt treatment of infections with appropriate antibiotics. 'Acyclovir' is very useful for herpetic infections. Patients with severe hypogammaglobulinaemia and recurrent infections may benefit from regular normal immunoglobulin injections. Fresh frozen plasma may be substituted if the patient cannot have i.m. injections because of thrombocytopenia.

Prognosis

1. Related to stage of disease.
2. Overall median survival six years.
3. Death usually associated with bone marrow failure or infection.
4. Acute transformation analogous to CGL is very rare.

T-cell chronic lymphocytic leukaemia (T-CLL).

Much less common than B CLL in United Kingdom. Generally greater splenomegaly for same stage of disease. May occur in younger age group.

PROLYMPHOCYTIC LEUKAEMIA

Less common than CLL.
May have B or T cell characteristics.
Diagnosis based on peripheral blood appearances and immunology — see
Table 9.1.

Clinical and laboratory features

1. Splenomegaly prominent.
2. Lymphadenopathy slight or absent.
3. Elderly males predominate.
4. Often very high WBC.

Treatment

1. Generally poor response to chemotherapy, but CHOP regime may be useful.
2. Splenectomy or splenic irradiation of possible benefit.
3. Leucapheresis may help if WBC very high.

Prognosis

Much worse than CLL.

HAIRY CELL LEUKAEMIA (leukaemic reticuloendotheliosis)

Typically 'hairy cells' are found in peripheral blood, but may not always be
apparent on light microscopy.

Clinical features

1. Usually elderly — male > female.
2. Pancytopenia.
3. Splenomegaly prominent.
4. Recurrent infections common.

Laboratory features

1. 'Hairy cells' — lymphocytes with spiky projections from cytoplasm.
2. Pancytopenia and especially monocytopenia.
3. Bone marrow aspiration often difficult. Usually hypocellular with lymphoid cells showing staining with tartrate resistant acid phosphatase.
4. Trephine biopsy often needed for diagnosis and shows excess fibrosis.

Treatment

1. Often unsatisfactory.
2. Splenectomy may improve pancytopenia and number of infections.
3. Typically chemotherapy is not helpful, but CHOP regime may produce some improvement.
4. Initial clinical trials have suggested that interferon treatment may be useful.

HTLV ASSOCIATED LEUKAEMIA

Recent work has shown that a virus subsequently named human T-cell lymphotrophic virus (HTLV) can be isolated from the T lymphocytes in certain T cell malignancies, predominantly in patients from Southern Japan and the Carribbean area.

Clinical and laboratory features

1. Affects adults of all ages.
2. In United Kingdom usually patients of West Indian origin.
3. Lymphadenopathy.
4. Skin lesions.
5. Bizarre T lymphocytes in the blood.
6. Hypercalcaemia.
7. High titres in blood of HTLVI antibody.

Treatment

Response to treatment is poor; usually rapidly downhill course.

SÉZARY SYNDROME

Leukaemic phase of *mycosis fungoides*, a T-cell lymphoma with intraepidermal skin involvement.

In Sézary syndrome, characteristic Sézary cells with convoluted nuclei appear in peripheral blood and the skin lesion tends to be a generalised erythroderma. Prognosis is poor.

REFERENCES

Bearman R B, Pangalis G A, Rappaport H 1978 Prolymphocytic leukaemia — clinical, histopathological and cytochemical observations. Cancer 42: 2360–2372
Bouroncle B A 1979 Leukaemic reticuloendotheliosis (hairy-cell leukaemia). Blood 53(3): 412–436
Goldman J M, Lu D P 1982 New approaches in chronic granulocytic leukaemia: origin prognosis and treatment. Seminars in Haematology 19: 241–256
Goldman J M, Preisler H D (eds) 1984 Leukaemias. Butterworth, London

20. MYELODYSPLASTIC SYNDROMES (MDS)

DEFINITION

A group of related disorders having the following features in common:
1. Dysplastic maturation of one or more haematological cell lines.
2. Variable cytopenias.
3. Propensity to transform into AML.

A variety of classifications of MDS have been suggested, none of which is entirely satisfactory. Disorders considered to be myelodysplastic syndromes include:
1. Preleukaemia: a general term applied to MDS; retrospectively many AML's have a prodromal MDS phase.
2. Refractory anaemia with or without excess of blasts.
3. Smouldering leukaemia: > 20% myeloblasts in marrow. Appearances may simulate acute myeloid leukaemia, however in smouldering leukaemia progression is very slow.
4. Chronic myelomonocytic leukaemia (CMML) sometimes considered as MDS, but better classified as a chronic leukaemia (p. 116).
5. Acquired primary sideroblastics anaemia (p. 15).

CLINICAL FEATURES

1. Usually elderly patients, but may develop in younger patients a few years after radiotherapy or alkylating agent therapy.
2. Anaemia (Ch. 1), leucopenia (Ch. 12) and thrombocytopenia (Ch. 11), either separately or together as a pancytopenia (Ch. 13).
3. Marked enlargement of liver, spleen or lymph nodes is *unusual*.
4. Transformation to acute myelomonocytic leukaemia is usual, however may not occur for many years.

INVESTIGATIONS

1. Blood count and film: variable cytopenias, agranular neutrophils with hypersegmented or hyposegmented (Pelger-Huet-like anomaly) nuclei. Mild oval macrocytosis. Relative or absolute monocytosis is common.
2. NAP score often low.
3. Haemoglobin electrophoresis — often shows high HbF level.
4. Marrow aspirate: commonly hypercellular with granulocyte series showing abnormal maturation and paucity of mature forms. Usually a small excess of blasts. The erythroid series shows megaloblastic-like changes often with ring sideroblasts. Occasionally increased fibrosis or hypocellularity is seen on trephine biopsy particularly when MDS is secondary to radiotherapy or cytotoxics.
5. Serum and urinary lysozyme are often increased.
6. Cytogenetics (on marrow aspirate): chromosome abnormalities are common, particularly monosomy 7 and fuzzy chromosomes. An abnormal karyotype indicates a worse prognosis.
7. Marrow culture investigations (in research centres): poor myeloid colony forming ability.

Management

1. Supportive treatment for particular cytopenia(s). See Chapter 15.
2. Conventional cytotoxic treatment is usually unsuccessful and dangerous. Efforts are now being directed at stimulating the dysplastic myeloid precursors to differentiate into functionally mature cells using chemical inducers such as ultra low dose cytosine arabinoside e.g. 20mg b.d. s.c. for 21 days or vitamin D analogues.

PROGNOSIS

Extremely variable. Many patients are elderly and will die of other diseases. In general the greater percentage of blasts in the marrow, the worse the prognosis.

REFERENCES

Bennett J M, Catovsky D, Daniel M T, Flandrin G, Galton D A G, Gralnick H R, Sultan C 1982 Proposals for the classification of the myelodysplastic syndromes. British Journal of Haematology 51: 189–199
Geary C G 1983 The diagnosis of pre-leukaemia. British Journal of Haematology 55: 1–6

21. MYELOMA

DEFINITION

Malignant proliferation of plasma cells associated with monoclonal immunoglobulin production and clinically complicated by bone lesions, marrow failure, immunoparesis and renal failure.

PRESENTING FEATURES

1. Usually elderly.
2. Recurrent bacterial infections.
3. Bone pain, pathological fractures.
4. Weight loss, anorexia, malaise.
5. Renal failure.
6. Symptomatic anaemia or bleeding from any site.
7. Unrelated clinical problem but persistently raised ESR or monoclonal band on protein electrophoresis or pancytopenia.
8. Symptoms of hypercalcaemia (see below).
9. Solitary soft-tissue or bony tumour (plasmacytoma).
10. Neurological abnormalities.
11. Hepatomegaly (30%), splenomegaly (10%) or lymphadenopathy (rare).

DIAGNOSTIC INVESTIGATIONS

1. Full blood count, platelet count and ESR.
2. Serum protein electrophoresis and immunoglobulin levels.
3. Early morning urine for Bence-Jones protein (free light chains).
4. Bone marrow aspiration, trephine biopsy if possible.
5. X-rays: chest, skull, pelvis, spine.
6. If needed surgical biopsy of soft-tissue, or accessible bony tumour.

DIFFERENTIAL DIAGNOSIS WITH BENIGN MONOCLONAL GAMMOPATHY (BMG)

One of the main problems in diagnosing the *early* case of myeloma is in distinguishing it from BMG. The following features favour myeloma:

1. Marrow plasma cells have abnormal morphology and constitute > 20% of nucleated cells.
2. Reduction in serum levels of normal immunoglobulins.
3. Paraprotein levels are > 35 G/l (IgG) or > 20 G/l (IgA).
4. Progressive increase in the level of the paraprotein.
5. Bence-Jones proteinuria present.
6. No clinical evidence of any underlying condition associated with BMG, e.g. carcinoma, chronic infection, auto-immune disease etc.

All patients with a presumptive diagnosis of BMG should be assessed yearly and not discharged from follow-up.

NB: The 'M' in 'M-band' stands for monoclonal, not myeloma or IgM.

BASELINE INVESTIGATIONS ONCE DIAGNOSIS OF MYELOMA IS ESTABLISHED

1. Blood: liver enzymes and bilirubin, uric acid, urea, electrolytes, creatinine, calcium, phosphate, albumin, total globulin.
2. 24 hour urine collection: quantitive assessment of calcium, total protein, Bence-Jones protein, creatinine clearance.
3. Plasma viscosity.
4. Coagulation screen (PT, TT, APTT, Fibrinogen).
5. Extended skeletal survey X-rays to include long bones and appropriate views to focus on any site of pain (bone scan not usually helpful).
6. MSU for microscopy and culture and other microbiological samples if any evidence of infection.

GENERAL MANAGEMENT

1. Urgent treatment of life-threatening complications.
2. Pain control.
3. Early liaison with radiotherapist.
4. Cytotoxic treatment of the tumour mass.
5. Mobilization and hydration.
6. Prevention and correction of other complications.
7. Psychological and social services support e.g. moving to ground floor flat, finding less strenuous job.

COMPLICATIONS OF MYELOMA

All the complications are manifestations of tumour activity, therefore the underlying aim is the treatment of the myeloma tumour mass.

Renal failure

Causes
1. Hypercalcaemia (dehydration, occasionally calculi).
2. Adult Fanconi's syndrome due to tubular damage by Bence-Jones protein.
3. Uric acid nephropathy.
4. Hyperviscosity syndrome (reduced renal perfusion).
5. Pre-renal ARF due to haemorrhage.
6. Occasionally analgesic nephropathy.
7. Increased incidence of urinary tract infections.
8. Direct renal damage due to infiltration by amyloid or myeloma cells.
9. Unrelated causes common to the age group e.g. prostatism, diabetes, hypertension.

Clinical features
Look for: distended bladder, signs of hyperviscosity, hyper- or hypotension, prostatic hypertrophy, signs of uraemia.

Investigations
1. Plasma: viscosity, calcium, uric acid, urea, creatinine, osmolality.
2. Urine: creatinine clearance, glucose testing, MSU, EMU for AFB, osmolality.
3. X-ray: plain abdomen, abdominal ultrasound, IVP (safe in myeloma provided no period of dehydration. Liaise closely with radiologist).

Treatment
1. Treat specific cause and established ARF or CRF in the usual ways.
2. Prevention:
   a. Encourage permanently adequate hydration to maintain daily urine output of > 2 litres
   b. Antibiotics for first signs of urinary tract infection
   c. Prompt treatment of hypercalcaemia
   d. Prevention of hyperuricaemia with allopurinol, 300 mg daily preferably starting forty-eight hours before each course of chemotherapy and continuing for at least two weeks.

NB: Serum uric acid will be raised in renal failure.

Bone lesions and bone pain

Clinical features

1. Pain very variable and not directly related to degree of X-ray abnormality. Can be constant and excruciating. Most commonly affected areas are vertebrae and ribs.
2. X-rays can show: diffuse/focal lytic lesions (in 60%), osteoporosis only (in 20%), normal bones (in 20%). Lysis most common with Bence-Jones myeloma (in 80%). Fractures, especially ribs. Vertebral compression.
3. May present acutely with long bone fracture.
4. Skull lytic lesions usually painless (c.f. similar lesions caused by carcinoma metastases).
5. Up to 10% of patients with myeloma have a solitary large, irregular, cystic bone tumour (plasmacytoma).
6. Patient may complain of bone tenderness, thoracic deformity, loss of height.

Investigations

1. Appropriate X-rays.
2. Alkaline phosphatase usually normal.

Treatment

Requires close liaison with radiotherapist and orthopaedic surgeon.

Preventative

1. Rapid, appropriate, cytotoxic treatment of the disease.
2. Encourage walking and gentle exercise. No heavy lifting.

Pain relief

1. Localized: radiotherapy alone often most useful.
2. Multi-focal: *effective* analgesia; doses to be titrated against the patients' pain; always to be given on a regular basis to anticipate recurrence of pain. There is no place for 'p.r.n.' analgesia in severe bone pain. For suggested analgesia regimes, see Chapter 24.

   Mithramycin 15 μ/kg dissolved in 500 ml 5% dextrose and given I.V. over four hours on each of two to four days. Halve the dose and number of doses in the presence of renal failure. (Main toxic effect: bleeding due to coagulopathy and thrombocytopenia.)
3. Pathological fracture of long bone: usually requires internal surgical fixation.
4. Indications for radiotherapy: local pain, pathological fractures (established and impending), spinal cord compression (requires urgent action), large soft tissue plasmacytoma.

Hypercalcaemia

Seen in 25% of myeloma patients at presentation.

Clinical features

Nausea, vomiting, constipation, polyuria, mental confusion. Metastatic calcification uncommon.

Investigations

1. Serum calcium
2. Serum albumin: often low, therefore need to correct calcium result (for every 1 g/l serum albumin is more than 46g/l subtract 0.022 mmol/l from calcium result. For every 1g/l serum albumin is less than 46g/dl add 0.022 mmol/l to calcium result).

Treatment (must be promptly dealt with)

1. Good analgesia to ensure mobilization. Correct dehydration, if necessary by intravenous fluids. If no response:
2. Corticosteroids: prednisolone 30–60 mg/ daily orally or hydrocortisone 160–240 mg/ daily iv. Usually only necessary for a few days. Taper to nil over three days as soon as calcium in normal range. If no response:
3. Phosphate, 1-2 g daily, orally, or lesser dose to limit of tolerance (diarrhoea). If no response:
4. Mithramycin (dose, see 'bone pain').
5. Calcitonin 4-8 units/kg daily SC.

Infection

Causes

1. Neutropenia (chemotherapy, infiltration of marrow).
2. Suppression of normal immunoglobulin production.

Clinical features

1. Usually bacterial, commonly pneumococcus or gram negative.
2. Commonly urinary tract or pneumonia.
3. Not particularly susceptible to viruses, except herpes zoster.
4. Full clinical examination required in a febrile patient.

Investigations

1. Neutrophilia as response to infection usually absent.
2. Before any antibiotic treatment started, take throat swab, MSU, sputum samples and three separate sets of blood cultures.

Treatment

1. Consult with microbiologist.
2. Parenteral antibiotics often needed for anything more than a trivial infection.
3. The patient with recurrent UTIs or bronchitis should keep antibiotics at home to start at first sign of infection.
4. Immunoglobulin therapy is usually ineffective.

Marrow failure

Causes
1. Usually marrow infiltration by myeloma.
2. Cytotoxic chemotherapy.

Clinical features
1. Anaemia common. Usually 7-9 g/dl and normochromic normocytic. Occasionally megaloblastic due to folate deficiency.
2. Severe thrombocytopenia uncommon. Rarely $< 50 \times 10^9/1$ and rarely symptomatic. Bleeding may also be due to coagulopathy (the M protein interacting with clotting factors).
3. Mild neutropenia (neutrophils 1.0–$2.0 \times 10^9/1$) common.

Investigations
1. Regular full blood counts and platelet counts.
2. Blood film may show leucoerythroblastic changes.
3. A few plasma cells may be found in the blood.
4. Marrow aspiration and biopsy occasionally necessary in differential diagnosis of pancytopenia due to the disease or chemotherapy, if due to therapy then usually hypoplastic.

Treatment
1. Bleeding in a thrombocytopenic patient will often require platelet transfusions (see Ch. 29).
2. Transfuse anaemic patients slowly with packed cells (*NB:* delay this in the patient with hyperviscosity syndrome until the hyperviscosity has been corrected as haematocrit is the single most important determinant of whole blood viscosity).

Hyperviscosity syndrome

Most commonly seen with an IgM paraprotein (i.e. Waldenström's macroglobulinaemia. IgM myeloma is extremely rare).

Clinical features
1. Eyes: visual disturbance of virtually any kind, at worst blindness. Flame retinal haemorrhages, dilation and tortuosity of veins, papilloedema.
2. Weakness, tiredness, anorexia.
3. Neurological: headache, dizzyness, nystagmus, confusion, coma, grand mal seizures, hearing loss, EEG changes.
4. Haematological: bleeding, particularly nose, GIT and urinary tract.

Investigations
1. ESR.
2. Whole blood and plasma viscosity. Normal plasma viscosity is approximately 1–2 cp, hyperviscosity syndrome usually seen > 4 cp.

Treatment

1. Ideally, referral to a specialist centre for plasmapheresis on cell separator, usually intensively for 1–2 days.
2. If referral impossible, bedside plasmapheresis can be achieved by bleeding patient of 500 ml into a citrated blood donor pack, spinning it down in a refrigerated centrifuge, taking off the plasma and transfusing red cells back into the patient with saline replacement. Repeat 1–2 times daily until symptoms improve. Even the removal of small amounts of plasma may be beneficial. Liaise with hospital blood bank.

Neurological abnormalities

Very variable, e.g.

1. Collapsed vertebrae causing spinal cord compression. Any sphincter disturbance or paretic neurological signs or symptoms require urgent spine X-ray and myelogram. Close liaison with radiotherapist and neuro-surgeon vital as cord compression requires urgent DXT and/or surgical decompression to prevent paraplegia.
2. Peripheral neuropathy (amyloid, uraemia, vincristine therapy).
3. Confusional states (uraemia, infection, hypercalcaemia, hyperviscosity, steroid therapy).
4. Cranial nerve lesions (myeloma deposits in bone at base of skull).

CHEMOTHERAPY FOR MYELOMA

Ideas are constantly changing and you should seek specialist advice. Currently useful:

First line drugs

1. Melphalan 5 mg/m^2 oral plus prednisolone 40 mg/m^2 oral daily, for 4–7 days, repeated every six weeks, or
2. Cyclophosphamide continuously 50–100 mg/day. Cross resistance does not necessarily occur.

Second line drugs

Vincristine, BCNU, Adriamycin, intravenous cyclophosphamide. While on cytotoxics for myeloma, a white cell count of 2–3 × $10^9/1$ and platelets of 50–150 × $10^9/1$ are common and are well tolerated. If a drop in the blood count is sudden and is thought to be due to the drugs rather than the disease, then reduce the dose of the next course rather than delay it.

REFERENCES

Salmon S E (ed) 1982 Myeloma and related disorders. Clinics in Haematology 11(1):

22. LYMPHOMAS

DEFINITION

Malignant tumours of lymphoid tissue of two main types:
1. Hodgkins Disease (HD).
2. Non-Hodgkins Lymphoma (NHL).

CLASSIFICATION

1. Hodgkins disease
   Classified histologically into 4 main types:
   a. Nodular sclerosis (may be subdivided in addition by cell predominance).
   b. Lymphocyte predominant.
   c. Mixed cellularity.
   d. Lymphocyte depleted.
2. Non-Hodgkins lymphoma
   Classification here is confusing and controversial and there are several available, based on morphological features and on lymphocyte physiology and immunology. Most are of B cell origin, with a few T cell tumours and true histiocytic types.

The main classifications in use at present are those of:
Rappaport
Kiel
Lukes and Collins
British National Lymphoma Investigation (BNLI)
Dorfman
WHO (World Health Organisation)

In addition a *Working Formulation for Clinical Usage* has recently been drawn up by the National Cancer Institute. Most classifications identify NHL in 3 main prognostic groups:
   a. Low grade malignancy.
   b. Intermediate malignancy.
   c. High grade malignancy.

This classification is based on:
  a. Cell type
  b. Pattern of involvement of the lymph node (nodular or dif-
     fuse).
Survival is significantly different in these groups and treatment is selected
accordingly.

CLINICAL FEATURES

1. Lymphadenopathy — usually painless, one or more regions.
2. Weight loss.
3. Fever (usually slight and showing diurnal fluctuation — classic
   Pel-Ebstein fever rare nowadays).
4. Sweats (especially at night).
5. Bone pain/back pain (especially in HD).
6. Fatigue, anorexia and other generalised symptoms.
7. Pruritus (especially HD).
8 Other skin lesions (subcutaneous nodules, erythroderma, ex-
   foliative dermatitis, mycosis fungoides, etc.).
9. Enlarged liver/spleen — spleen size not necessarily related to
   involvement in HD.
10. Jaundice.
11. Symptoms and signs of anaemia.
12. Opportunistic infections, especially viral, TB, fungi (i.e. depen-
    dent on cell mediated immunity), or bacterial (in association
    with hypogammaglobulinaemia or neutropenia).
13. Alcohol induced pain (rare, occurs in HD).
14. CNS symptoms and signs (papilloedema, headache, nerve pal-
    sies — suggest CNS infiltration. More common in NHL).
15. Waldeyer's ring enlargement (NHL).
16. Localised symptoms related to site, e.g. GI tract, respiratory.

STAGING

There is universal agreement about clinical and pathological staging accord-
ing to the Ann Arbor classification:
  Stage I: one or more contiguous groups of nodes, on same side of
             diaphragm.
  Stage II: two or more separate nodal groups on same side of diaphragm.
  Stage III: nodal disease on both sides of diaphragm.
  Stage IV: metastatic extranodal spread outwith lymphoid system (e.g.
             liver, marrow, lung, CNS, etc.).
S as a suffix denotes splenic disease. E denotes isolated extranodal disease as
the prime site without widespread involvement of lymph nodes, or localised
extension of disease from lymph nodes into adjacent soft tissue e.g. isolated
involvement of a part of bowel with only contiguous nodes involved.

Symptoms

Patients in all groups may show cardinal symptoms which are:

1. Weight loss > 10% total body weight in preceeding six months.
2. Unexplained fever > 38°C.
3. Night sweats sufficient to require change of night clothes. Presence of any of the above symptoms is denoted by the suffix B; and absence by the suffix A, e.g. Stage IIA, IIIB, IIS, etc.

Importance of accurate staging:

1. *Hodgkins disease.*

   Treatment of all detectable disease at the time of presentation with a view to cure is the aim. Spread of disease is predictable between nodal groups and prognosis and type of treatment is highly dependent on stage. Hence accurate staging is *essential.*

2. *Non Hodgkins lymphoma.*

   As a whole these tumours are less curable than H.D., and prognosis and type of treatment is more related to histological type than stage. Some types of tumour have intrinsically more likelihood of widespread involvement at diagnosis, yet remain of overall relatively benign course. Hence full staging is not always essential.

INVESTIGATIONS

Involves:

1. Establishing histological diagnosis.
2. Staging extent of disease.

Lymph node biopsy

If choice available, preferably not inguinal as there is a high incidence of non-specific reactive changes. Imprints from fresh tissue useful for cytology. Marker studies may be carried out on fresh tissue — especially relevant in NHL, e.g. T or B cell origin. May need rebiopsy if diagnosis in doubt first time.

Blood investigations

1. *Full blood count*

   Look for evidence of marrow involvement or failure. Neutrophilia and eosinophilia seen in HD.

   May be lymphocytosis with lymphomatous cells in blood in NHL.

2. *Liver function tests*

   May show evidence of parenchymal involvement or biliary obstruction from enlarged nodes. Not a very reliable indicator of liver involvement however. Plasma protein electrophoresis and quantitative immunoglobulins.

Diffuse increase in immunoglobulins sometimes in HD and in some NHL.
3. *Direct antiglobulin (Coombs) test*
   Auto-immune haemolysis common especially in NHL.
4. *Routine renal function*
   Baseline for treatment. May be abnormal if obstructive uropathy or renal infiltration.
5. *Uric acid*
6. *Bone chemistry*
   Raised alkaline phosphatase or calcium may suggest bone involvement.
   Some T cell NHL present with hypercalcaemia.

Bone marrow aspirate and trephine biopsy

To assess marrow involvement plus cellularity. Trephine essential — ideally from two or more sites.

Radiological

1. *Chest X-ray:*
   Hilar or mediastinal nodes
   Lung infiltration.
2. *Abdominal lymphography:*
   Outline pelvic, iliac and para-aortic nodes
   Allows identification of abnormal nodes for further biopsy in HD
   Useful for follow-up as dye remains in nodes for up to six months
   Less routinely used since advent of CT scanning.
3. *Computed tomography (CT scan):*
   To some extent superseded lymphography.
   Very useful for detecting lymph nodes in porta hepatis.
4. *Ultrasound scan:*
   For liver, splenic and nodal involvement — increasingly useful as atraumatic and repeatable.
5. *Abdominal lymphoscintigraphy:*
   Isotopic outline of nodes as alternative to lymphography.
6. *Bone scan:*
   Not usually routine but perform if symptoms suggestive of bony involvement.

Investigations for selected patients

1. *Liver biopsy:*
   Closed liver biopsy is of limited use as it is easy to miss isolated lesions
   An open biopsy at laparotomy or laparoscopy gives better results.

2. *Staging laparotomy:*
In HD accurate staging essential in order to eradicate disease in all affected areas. Therefore staging laparotomy usually performed on patients with stage I, II and IIIA disease. Only justified if it will potentially alter treatment regime, and there is increasing evidence that it may be unnecessary. Includes:
   a. Splenectomy (thereby eliminating need to irradiate spleen)
   b. Wedge liver biopsies from both lobes plus needle biopsies from both lobes
   c. Biopsy of any suspicious or selected representative nodes
   d. In females of reproductive age — oophoropexy to shift ovaries out of potential radiation fields.

Patients with stage IIIB or IV are almost certain to receive chemotherapy rather than radiotherapy as their definitive treatment and hence laparotomy is unnecessary.

In NHL accurate staging is less essential, so justification for laparotomy is seldom present.
3. Specific examination of Waldeyer's ring.
4. GI tract: barium studies, endoscopy and biopsy if indicated.

TREATMENT

1. *Radiotherapy:*
Used to achieve cure in localised disease, or as palliation in bulk disease, or when specific problems occur with local node involvement, e.g. jaundice from porta hepatis node enlargement.
2. *Chemotherapy:*
May be curative or palliative. Single agent chemotherapy is seldom indicated in HD as never curative and prejudices more radical combination regimes. Most regimes for H.D. are four drug combinations. In NHL, chemotherapy is more varied, ranging from single agents to combinations of five or more drugs.

Hodgkins Disease

Selection of treatments

Aim in newly diagnosed patients is *cure*. Treatment must obviously be individually tailored to the patient but in general can be summarised as:

Stage I, II: radical radiotherapy
Stage IIIA: radiotherapy ± chemotherapy
Stage IIIB, IV: chemotherapy

Localised extranodal disease e.g. bone, lung — radiotherapy and chemotherapy.

Lymphocyte depletion with B symptoms any stage: include chemotherapy.

Radiotherapy fields
Extended fields are treated with 35–40 Gy over approximately four week interval.
1. For supradiaphragmatic disease:
'Mantle' area (includes all nodes above diaphragm and upper para-aortics).
2. For infradiaphragmatic disease:
'Inverted Y' area (includes para-aortic, iliac and pelvic nodes).
3. For stage III disease:
'Total nodal' area.
Treatment always extends beyond the point of known disease spread. Splenic area should be irradiated if spleen is not removed.

Problems of radiotherapy
1. Nausea and vomiting (anti-emetics should be used generously).
2. Bone marrow suppression.
3. Skin damage and alopecia.
4. Lung fibrosis.
5. Sterility.

Chemotherapy
Main regimes (for details of drugs see Ch. 23):
MOPP — mustine, vincristine (Oncovin), procarbazine, prednisolone.
MVPP — mustine, vinblastine, procarbazine, prednisolone.
CHVPP — chlorambucil, vinblastine, procarbazine, prednisolone.
ABVD — Adriamycin, bleomycin, vinblastine, dacarbazine (DTIC).
MOPP and MVPP are the classic and still widely used regimes. Both have the problems of severe mustine-induced vomiting and hence CHVPP was introduced with chlorambucil as a substitute. The efficacy of CHVPP in the long term is still being assessed. ABVD is largely confined to relapsed patients.
Problems of chemotherapy are similar to radiotherapy.
A minimum of six courses of treatment, each separated by four to six weeks, is usual.
Combined chemo and radiotherapy probably increases chances of cure but this has to be weighed against problems of intractable bone marrow toxicity and substantial risk of second malignancies.

Non Hodgkins Lymphoma

Radiotherapy
Usually palliative
1. Moderate doses to bulk disease.
2. Low dose total body irradiation at weekly intervals as alternative to chemotherapy.
3. In occasional patients with very localised disease, radical radiotherapy may be curative.

Chemotherapy

Usually palliative but may induce long term remission. Curability is greatest paradoxically in certain high grade but localised lymphomas such as immunoblastic or true histiocytic types.

Low grade lymphomas are often widely disseminated but compatible with long term survival, and may not even require treatment initially.

Main regimes (for details of drugs see Ch. 23):

    1. Low grade lymphoma — chlorambucil ± prednisolone.
    2. Intermediate grade lymphoma — COP (cyclophosphamide, vincristine, prednisolone).
    3. High grade lymphoma — CHOP (cyclophosphamide, adriamycin, vincristine, prednisolone). M-BACOP (methotrexate, bleomycin, adriamycin, cyclophosphamide, vincristine, prednisolone).

Newer regimes may include vindesine, cytosine arabinoside, and etoposide, all of which show activity against lymphoma.

At least six courses are usually given; the number necessary to induce a remission then an additional two or three. Maintenance therapy is sometimes used, but its role in prolonging survival is uncertain.

In HD and NHL, after remission is obtained, re-assessment can be carried out by repeating initially abnormal investigations e.g., marrow trephine, CAT scanning.

In NHL it is often difficult to decide how intensively to pursue treatment in the less curable groups. More aggressive regimes may yet result in better cure rates, especially if radical techniques such as autologous or allogeneic bone marrow transplantation are implemented.

CNS disease is increasingly a problem in NHL. Intrathecal chemotherapy and cranial irradiation may be effective in established cases. Prophylactic CNS therapy (analogous to ALL) has a place in certain high grade tumours with high CNS relapse rates (e.g. lymphoblastic lymphoma).

PROGNOSIS

Related to *stage* and *histology* in HD, and largely to *histology* in NHL.

    1. *HD*
        Stage IA, IIA: 90% potentially cured with radiotherapy.
        Stage IIIB, IV: 30–40% four year survival with chemotherapy.
    2. *NHL*
        Low grade: median survival, five years.
        Intermediate grade: median survival, two to three years.
        High grade: median survival, 12 months.

Long term problems
1. Relapse — treatment becomes increasingly difficult and cure is unlikely.
2. Bone marrow toxicity — extensive treatment may compromise marrow permanently.
3. Immunosuppression.
4. Second malignancies (commonly AML induced by treatment — especially with a combination of chemotherapy and radiotherapy).
5. Sterility (consider sperm banking prior to treatment).

REFERENCES

Kaplan H S 1981 Hodgkin's disease — biology, treatment and prognosis. Blood 57: 813–822
McElwain T J 1984 Curable cancers: Hodgkin's disease and non-Hodgkin's lymphomas. British Journal of Hospital Medicine 31: 10–19
Rosenberg S A, Kaplan H S 1982 Malignant lymphomas: aetiology, immunology, pathology and treatment. Academic Press, London

23. CYTOTOXIC CHEMOTHERAPY

GENERAL GUIDELINES

1. Almost without exception, the drugs used have wide-ranging and sometimes serious unwanted effects — the difference between a therapeutic dose and a lethal dose may be very small. Commonly these drugs are prescribed by senior doctors but administered by junior doctors and it is vital that the latter familiarise themselves with the appropriate doses, routes of administration and unwanted effects.

2. Try to arrange treatment in your unit so that patients get to know one or two doctors well and do not have to be treated by a different houseman each week.

3. The most convenient way of giving multiple intravenous injections is via a butterfly steel needle — a plastic cannula is more painful and an ordinary venepuncture needle is awkward to use. The tubing attached to the butterfly needle allows for easy handling of the syringe and facilitates giving successive syringefuls of drugs.

4. Make sure that the patients arm is comfortably supported (e.g. resting on a pillow) before beginning the injection.

5. Pay strict attention to aseptic technique.

6. Take great care when preparing the drugs for injection. Avoid spillage and wear gloves and goggles. Wash off any drug spilled onto your skin. Although toxic effects of very small contaminating doses of these drugs have not been established it is wise to take precautions.

7. Certain intravenous drugs — BCNU, vincristine, vindesine, vinblastine, adriamycin, daunorubicin, DTIC and mustine cause severe tissue necrosis if extravasated. Therefore these drugs should not be injected directly into a vein but should be injected slowly (over 5 min) through the rubber injection site of a fast running saline drip (a butterfly needle can still be used). Never start injecting these drugs unless you are sure that you

have a good clean venepuncture and stop immediately if you suspect that the drip has tissued. After injecting the drugs allow 20ml or so of saline to run in so that you do not risk spreading the drug along the withdrawn needle track and to ensure that the full dose has been given intravenously.

If you knowingly extravasate one of these drugs then infiltrate the affected tissues with saline to dilute the irritant effect. Many of the drug manufacturers also recommend infiltration of the site with hyaluronidase or hydrocortisone.

8. Familiarise yourself with those intravenous drugs that are quite harmless if extravasated (any drug that can be given i.m. or subcutaneously will apply) as it will save needless worry if the drip should tissue. These include cytosine arabinoside, methotrexate, cyclophosphamide and asparaginase.

9. Most cytotoxic injections damage the vein lining to some degree therefore it is wise to rotate usage of veins week by week instead of always using the same one. Many leukaemic patients have so many venepunctures that they end up with only one or two usable veins and these are often very tiny. If you are not highly competent at venepuncture, then do not practice on these patients but instead ask for help from someone who is more experienced.

10. Beware of mixing syringes up when giving intravenous therapy to a succession of patients at the end of a busy clinic. If you have to prepare the injections in bulk, always clearly mark each syringe with a glass-writing pen. Never just lay the syringe out with the original vial beside it as sole means of identification.

11. Remember to check the platelet count before giving any intramuscular injections — the critical level varies from patient to patient but an i.m. injection in a patient with a platelet count of less than $40 \times 10^9/1$ will often produce a painful haematoma.

12. Doses are ideally calculated in terms of the body surface area (i.e. per metre^2) as this is more directly proportional to circulating blood volume than per kilogram body weight. Slide rule nomograms to calculate m^2 are available from many drug companies.

13. Know the timing of the peak myelosuppressive effect of the drugs that you are giving so that you can plan blood counts sensibly. Drugs that do not cause dose-limiting myelosuppression are vincristine, asparaginase, bleomycin and steroids.

14. Some cytotoxic drugs are very expensive (e.g. adriamycin, vindesine, and asparaginase all cost more than £50 for a single dose) and care should be taken that they are not wasted.

15. A useful working classification of cytotoxic drugs:
   a. Alkylating agents (mustine, busulphan, cyclophosphamide, melphalan, chlorambucil)
   b. Antimetabolites (methotrexate, cytosine arabinoside, 6-mercaptopurine, 6-thioguanine)
   c. Vinca alkaloids (vincristine, vinblastine, vindesine)
   d. Anti-mitotic antibiotics (daunorubicin, adriamycin, mithramycin, bleomycin)
   e. Miscellaneous (asparaginase, BCNU, CCNU, procarbazine).
16. The more aggressive haematological malignancies are generally treated by a 'cocktail' of the above drugs i.e. combination chemotherapy. The rationale behind this method of treatment is to attack the malignant cell by several methods at once (the drugs above having different modes of action) and to minimise specific toxic side effects of individual drugs. Often these chemotherapy schedules are referred to by a mnemonic consisting of the first letters of the drugs used
   e.g. DAT — Daunorubicin, cytosine, Arabinoside, Thioguanine: CHOP — Cyclophosphamide, Hydroxydaunorubicin (adriamycin), Oncovin (vincristine), Prednisolone.

Unwanted effects

Many patients are frightened of intravenous cytotoxic therapy, particularly if they have experienced unpleasant side effects with previous treatment. The best way of reassuring the patient is by anticipating and preventing side effects where possible (e.g. anti-emetics). Those side-effects that cannot be prevented, e.g. alopecia, should be explained to the patient before the treatment starts.

Alopecia
Seen with adriamycin, daunorubicin, vincristine, and high dose cyclophosphamide. Trials are currently being carried out on cooling the scalp with ice packs to prevent alopecia, but there is no other preventative measure known at the moment. It is vital to warn the patient of the possibility of hair loss and reassure them that, should it be necessary, they can be supplied with a good wig at short notice. Cytotoxic induced alopecia always recovers, although sometimes only after some months.

Nausea and vomiting
The degree of disturbance varies greatly with different drugs and with different patients. Drugs especially liable to cause vomiting are Adriamycin, mustine, high dose cyclophosphamide and BCNU.

Prophylactic anti-emetics should be given with these and the patient warned.

The mechanisms of cytotoxic-induced vomiting are poorly understood but include direct action on gastro-intestinal motility with or without direct action on the brain-stem vomiting centre. Some of the nausea experienced is, understandably, of psychological origin either because of general anxiety about the injection or because of previous reactions to the drug. Reassurance and understanding on the doctor's part play a significant role in reducing symptoms but the skilled manipulation of anti-emetics and/or sedatives is even more useful. The patient and doctor should work together at what is best in each case — some patients prefer to have an empty stomach, others prefer to have eaten recently. If nausea persists at home, then anti-emetics should be prescribed to be taken routinely and not on a p.r.n. basis.

It is not helpful to give oral anti-emetics to a vomiting patient. Intramuscular preparations can be given if the platelet count allows but, often more useful, is a suppository. All anti-emetics can be specially made up in suppository form by the hospital pharmacist and this is often a very good way of giving them. If possible start all anti-emetics an hour before the cytotoxics are given. They all have a sedative effect to some degree and patients should know before they come up to the clinic that they should not drive themselves home and should be accompanied on public transport. There is, unfortunately, no single 'wonder drug' anti-emetic that will work in every patient but one of the following schedules will usually be helpful (adult doses have been given here):

(i)   Chlorpromazine
       i.m. :   12.5–50mg   8 hourly p.r.n.
       Oral :   25–50 mg   8 hourly p.r.n.
       p.r. :   100mg suppository 8 hourly p.r.n.
(ii) Prochlorperazine (Stemetil)
       i.m. :   12.5mg   4–8 hourly p.r.n.
       Oral :   10mg   4–8 hourly p.r.n.
       up.r. :   25mg suppository 4–8 hourly p.r.n.
(iii) Metoclopramide (Maxalon)
       i.m., oral, i.v.: 10–20 mg 4–8 hourly p.r.n.
(iv) For in-patients or selected out-patients who have responsible supervision at home, lorazepam 3mg orally or i.v. can be given in addition to an anti-emetic. It has an amnesic and sedative action and the patient, although rousable (and therefore will wake up to vomit and not inhale vomitus) will sleep soundly for up to 16 hours after treatment and will wake up with little memory of the anxiety and nausea.

(v) Studies are currently being carried out on various new compounds with anti-emetic properties. These include methylprednisolone and the cannabinoids. One of the latter is available for clinical use — nabilone 1–2mg p.o. twice daily. Metaclopramide, mentioned in iii. above, is claimed by some investigators to be more effective in greater doses than those conventionally used — up to 100mg — though these higher doses have a higher incidence of dystonic reactions.

Mouth ulcers
Seen particularly with methotrexate, daunorubicin and Adriamycin. Symptomatic relief can be obtained with benzocaine lozenges, xylocaine viscous gel or choline salicylate dental paste (Bonjela, Teejel). Folinic acid used as a mouthwash may be effective when the cause has been methotrexate therapy.

Teratogenicity
There is an increased risk of congenital abnormalities in children born to parents receiving cytotoxic chemotherapy. Patients should be advised to employ contraception. In many patients undergoing treatment for malignant disease though, the problem does not arise as libido and fertility are often greatly reduced. Pregnant women who need cytotoxic chemotherapy pose a very special problem and specialised advice should be sought. Young men who need chemotherapy may have their semen preserved frozen in a sperm bank for later use by artificial insemination.

Anaphylaxis
Acute anaphylactic reactions are possible with any of the parenteral cytotoxics, but are particularly common with asparaginase. Do not begin the injection without checking that adrenaline, hydrocortisone and chlorpheniramine are at hand and that resuscitation equipment is within reasonable distance.

INDIVIDUAL CYTOTOXIC DRUGS

For each drug the approved name, proprietary name, and shortened name in common usage (if any) are given. The drugs have been listed alphabetically:

ASPARAGINASE (COLASPASE) Crasnitin, Erwinia

Routes of administration
Usually given intravenously as an infusion in saline over half an hour or as a slow i.v. bolus over 5 minutes.

Main haematological uses
ALL, Lymphomas. Occasionally, AML (M5 and M3, p.   ).

Typical dose used
1000–4000 units/m^2 daily for 5 to 14 days.

Timing of peak fall in blood count
Virtually no myelosuppression.

Main unwanted effects
1. Anaphylaxis is common. A test dose must be given before treatment with asparaginase, particularly when resuming treatment after an interval (details below).
2. It is toxic to many systems and damage reported includes renal toxicity, hepatic damage, pancreatic malfunction with hyperglycaemia or pancreatitis, somnolence, extrapyramidal symptoms and signs, and coagulopathy with reduced fibrinogen and factor V.
3. Rarely, alopecia, nausea.

Practical points in administration
1. It does not irritate the skin.
2. Test dose: make up a solution of asparaginase so that you have approximately 50 units in 0.5 ml of saline. Inject this intracutaneously on the volar aspect of the forearm. Observe the site 3 hours later if there is any evidence of a local inflammatory/ allergic response then it is not safe to give asparaginase to that patient. The two preparations of asparaginase are immunologically distinct, so the other formulation may then be tried, though a test dose should be performed with that too.

BCNU (CARMUSTINE)   BiCNU

Routes of administration
i.v. only, added to a saline or dextrose drip and usually given over two hours. BCNU has a low liquefying point (27°C) therefore discard any vial found to be liquid.

Main haematological use
Second line treatment in myeloma, lymphomas.

Typical dose used
200 mg/m^2 i.v. infusion, once or twice every 6 weeks.

Timing of peak fall in blood count
Delayed marrow suppression. Nadir of platelet count at 4–5 weeks, nadir of white cell count at 5–6 weeks.

Main unwanted effects
1. Dose limiting marrow suppression.
2. Acute nausea and vomiting common.
3. Reversible elevation of liver enzymes.

Practical points in administration
1. Nausea can be minimised by giving half the dose on two successive days. Anti-emetic virtually always needed. Vomiting will start within two hours and may last for 6–8 hours.
2. Not normally given more frequently than every 6 weeks.
3. The reconstituted solution will remain stable for 48 hours at 4°C.

BLEOMYCIN

Routes of administration
Given i.m., i.v., i.a., subcutaneous, intrapleural, intraperitoneal. Usually given intravenously as an infusion or slow push injection in saline 5–200 ml.

Main haematological use
Lymphomas.

Typical dose used
15 mg weekly i.v.

Timing of peak fall in blood count
It is not normally myelosuppressive so does not usually affect the blood count.

Main unwanted effects
1. 50% of patients develop stomatitis.
   This is often the best guide to individual tolerance to the drug.
2. 50% of patients develop skin rashes, probably related to the total cumulative dose and not usually apparent until 150 mg or so have been given. They can take the form of increased pigmentation, light sensitivity, hyperkeratosis, or tender swollen finger tips.
3. Lung toxicity is common and is virtually always seen once the cumulative dose is over 300 mg. 1% of patients on bleomycin develop fatal pulmonary fibrosis and 10% of patients receiving less than 300 mg total dose will develop pneumonitis. The symptoms are dyspnoea (often severe) and non-productive cough, and bilateral crepitations are heard. The chest x-ray in the pneumonitic stage will show patchy opacities, usually in the lower fields. Pulmonary damage is worsened by previous or concurrent radiotherapy to the lungs.
4. There may be a histamine-like reaction to the injection with a rise in blood pressure, hot flushes and fever. This is self limiting but very frightening for the patient.
5. Rarely, there may be an acute anaphylactoid reaction to the injection which is treated in the usual manner i.e. Piriton 10–20 mg slow i.v., hydrocortisone 100–200 mg i.v., 0.5 ml of 1 in 1000 adrenaline subcutaneously, and volume expansion with i.v. fluids if necessary.

6. The injection site may be painful even with no extravasation.
7. Nausea and vomiting common.
8. Alopecia frequent.

Practical points in administration

1. While on treatment, do a weekly chest x-ray and abandon treatment at the first sign of lung changes. Take any pulmonary symptoms very seriously. Severe pneumonitis is occasionally irreversible but it may respond to high-dose steroids plus a broad-spectrum antibiotic. Changes in pulmonary function during bleomycin treatment are best followed by measurement of the vital capacity.
2. If the serum creatinine is more than 180 mmol/l give 50% of the planned dose. If the creatinine is more than 360 mmol/l then do not administer bleomycin.
3. Anti-emetics will usually be needed.
4. Warn about alopecia.

BUSULPHAN   Myleran

Routes of administration
Oral only: white tablets of 0.5 mg and 2 mg.

Main haematological use
CGL, polycythaemia rubra vera, primary thrombocythaemia.

Typical dose used
2–4 mg daily, sometimes continuously for over 2 years. Occasionally used as a pulsed stat dose, e.g. 100 mg every 6 weeks.

Timing of peak fall in blood count
Up to six weeks.

Main unwanted effects

1. Marrow suppression, particularly platelets.
2. Dose dependent pulmonary fibrosis usually only evident after several years of treatment.
3. 5–10% show an increase in melanin pigmentation. Rarely Addison's sydrome develops.
4. In pre-menopausal women: ovarian suppression with amenorrhoea and menopausal symptoms. In men: azoospermia with sterility, testicular atrophy.

Practical points in administration

1. Warn appropriate patients about infertility.
2. In CGL discontinue treatment with busulphan once the white cell count has fallen to $10–15 \times 10^9/1$ and/or the platelet count has fallen to $100 \times 10^9/1$. Busulphan will continue to exert a myelosuppressive effect for up to 6 weeks after treatment has been stopped and irreversible marrow hypoplasia may ensue. Increased marrow reticulin may be associated with increased sensitivity to busulphan myelosuppression.

LOMUSTINE   CCNU

Routes of administration
Oral only: 40 mg blue capsules, 10 mg blue/white capsules.

Main haematological use
Second line treatment in some lymphomas.

Typical dose used
20–100 mg/m^2 as a single dose every 6–8 weeks.

Timing of peak fall in blood count
Platelet count radiv at 4 weeks, neutrophil count radiv at 6 weeks.

Main unwanted effects
1. Dose limiting marrow suppression. Occasionally irreversible.
2. Nausea and vomiting are very common. This usually starts within 4 hours of the dose and can continue for 24–48 hours.
3. Occasional transient elevation of liver enzymes.

Practical points in administration
1. Myelosuppression may occasionally be cumulative and therefore more profound with each treatment. The platelet count is usually worst affected.
2. Anti-emetics virtually always needed.
3. There is cross resistance with other nitrosoureas, but not with other alkylating agents.

CHLORAMBUCIL   Leukeran

Routes of administration
Oral only: yellow tablets of 2 mg and 5 mg.

Main haematological uses
CLL, Waldenstrom's, some lymphomas.

Typical doses used
Variable, e.g. 2–5 mg daily for 3–6 weeks or pulse treatment, e.g. 30 mg daily for three days each month.

Timing of peak fall in blood count
10 days to 3 weeks, then a further 2 weeks for recovery.

Main unwanted effects
1. Myelosuppression, particularly platelets. This may occasionally be irreversible on stopping the drug. Lymphopenia.
2. Rarely: nausea, alopecia, dermatitis, hepatotoxity, lung damage, peripheral neuropathy, fits.

CYCLOPHOSPHAMIDE   Endoxana

Routes of administration
Oral: white tablets of 10 mg, 50 mg; i.v. vials of 100 mg, 200 mg, 500 mg 1 g,
as a slow intravenous injection. Compatible with saline or 5% dextrose.
Non-irritant if extravasated.

Main haematological uses
A wide range of uses, e.g. myeloma, CLL, ALL, lymphomas and Hodgkin's
disease. Also used as an immunosuppressive in auto-immune disease.

Typical dose used
Very variable — from 10 mg orally up to stat i.v. doses of more than 1 g.
Doses of several grams are used to ablate recipients marrow before bone
marrow transplantation.

Timing of peak fall in blood count
5–10 days. Recovery starts at about the 14th day and is usually complete by
28th day.

Main unwanted effects
1. Nausea and vomiting, sometimes diarrhoea.
2. Haemorrhagic sterile cystitis with dysuria, frequency and haematuria. Long term: irreversible bladder fibrosis.
3. Alopecia. Usually complete with high intermittent doses, seen in
   20% of patients of doses of more than 100 mg daily. Usually
   evident 3 weeks after first treatment but often regrows by 3
   months even if still on treatment.
4. Immunosuppressive and moderately myelosuppressive. Platelets
   are relatively spared.

Practical points in administration
1. Warn the patient about possible hair loss.
2. To try and prevent sterile cystitis, the patient must maintain a
   high fluid intake; with high doses (over 200 mg daily or stat) the
   patient must drink at least 3 litres over the ensuring 24 hours.
   Doses used for marrow transplantation require forced diuresis
   and urine alkalinisation. Mesna, a relatively new drug, may help
   in the prevention of cystitis by preventing formation of the
   metabolites of cyclophosphamide that are particularly irritant to
   the bladder.
3. Cyclophosphamide reduces the hypoglycaemic affect of insulin
   and oral hypoglycaemic agents.
4. Cyclophosphamide potentiates suxamethonium — non-
   depolarising muscle relaxants should be used instead.

CYTOSINE ARABINOSIDE   Cytosar

Routes of administration
i.v., i.m., s.c., inthrathecal. May be given intravenously as a slow injection or
by infusion. For inthrathecal use the accompanying diluent solution should
NOT be used as it contains an irritant preservative. Use saline BP as diluent
instead.

Main haematological uses
AML, ALL, some use in lymphomas.

Typical dose used
100–150 mg/m^2

Timing of peak fall in blood count
5–7 days with a further 10–20 days for recovery.

Main unwanted effects
1. Marked myelosuppression in over 60% of cases.
2. Muscle weakness.
3. Nausea and vomiting in approximately 15% of patients. Constipation.
4. Marked immunosuppression.
5. Occasionally: oral ulceration, hypersensitivity, renal or hepatic
   damage.

Practical points in administration
1. Non-irritant if extravasated.

DAUNORUBICIN (RUBIDOMYCIN)   Cerubicin

Routes of administration
i.v. only, diluted in saline.

Main haematological uses
AML, ALL.

Typical dose used
40 mg/m^2 stat i.v. weekly or on two or three successive days.

Timing of peak fall in blood count
10–15 days.

Main unwanted effects
1 Cardiotoxicity, dependent on the total cumulative dose. Maximum safe total cumulative dose of the order of 500–600 mg/m^2.
   See doxorubicin section.
2. Alopecia.
3. Marked myelosuppression.
4. Nausea and vomiting.

Practical points in administration
1. Severe tissue damage if extravasated (see general notes).
2. Warn the patient about alopecia.

DOXORUBICIN (HYDROXYDAUNORUBICIN) Adriamycin

Routes of administration
i.v. only.

Main haematological uses
ALL, AML, Lymphomas.

Typical dose used
40–80 mg/m^2 as a single dose every 3–4 weeks.

Timing of peak fall in blood count
10–12 days.

Main unwanted effects
1. Cardiotoxicity. Incidence 0.25–10% when total cumulative dose of 550 mg/m^2 is reached. The risk of cardiotoxicity has to be weighed against the haematological necessity of continuing treatment beyond this dose. Cardiotoxicity usually takes the form of sudden death or intractable cardiac failure. It is usually impossible to predict, but may be heralded by persistant tachycardia or minor non-specific ECG changes.
2. Alopecia very common.
3. Nausea and vomiting common; sometimes diarrhoea.
4. Myelosuppression + + particularly neutrophils but is relatively short lasting, predictable and non-cumulative. Stomatitis.

Practical points in administration
1. Increased risk of cardiotoxicity with concurrent uncontrolled hypertension, congestive cardiac failure, simultaneous treatment with cyclophosphamide, previous mediastinal radiotherapy.
2. Reduce the dose in the presence of abnormal liver function tests, particularly those indicating obstructive jaundice. If bilirubin is 35–50 mmol/l, reduce dose by 50%, if bilirubin is more than 50 mmol/l then reduce dose by 75%.
3. Warn the patient about alopecia.
4. Warn the patient that for 24 hours or so after the injection they may pass red urine and notice red staining of saliva and tears.
5. Never give Adriamycin into the tubing of a drip containing heparin as it will be precipitated. It also reacts with hydrocortisone, dexamethasone, cephalothin and aminophylline.
6. Recommended total cumulative dose should not exceed 550 mg/m^2 (450 mg/m^2 if combined with cyclophosphamide therapy or thoracic irradiation).
7. Severe damage if extravasated.

MELPHALAN   Alkeran

Routes of administration
Oral: pink tablets of 2 mg and 5 mg.
i.v., i.a.; also used for tumour perfusion.

Main haematological uses
Myeloma.

Typical dose used
5–20 mg daily orally for 4–7 days, repeated every 4–6 weeks.

Timing of peak fall in blood count
3–4 weeks.

Main unwanted effects
  1. Nausea and vomiting.
  2. Bladder toxicity.
  3. Myelosuppression.
  4. Reduce dose or duration of treatment in the presence of renal failure.

6-MERCAPTOPURINE   Purinethol

Routes of administration
Oral only: beige tablets of 10 mg and 50 mg.

Main haematological uses
ALL, AML.

Typical dose used
100–200 mg/m^2 per day.

Timing of peak fall in blood count
2–3 weeks.

Main unwanted effects
  1. Myelosuppression.
  2. Hepatotoxic.
  3. Rarely: nausea, vomiting, oral ulceration.

Practical points of administration
  1. If being given concurrently with allopurinol, only give 25% of the normal 6-MP dose (6-MP is inactivated by xanthine oxidase which is itself inactivated by allopurinol).
  2. Monitor liver function tests.
  3. There is cross resistance with 6-MP and 6-thioguanine.
  4. Potent immunosuppressant.

METHOTREXATE   **Methotrexate**

Routes of administration
Oral: orange tablets of 2.5 mg.
i.v., i.a., i.t., i.m. Use normal saline as diluent.
Given as infusion or slow i.v. injection.

Main haematological uses
ALL, treatment and prophylaxis of meningeal leukaemia, lymphomas.

Typical doses used
Very variable. There are many current treatment schedules that involve
giving high doses (e.g. 500 mg intravenously) followed by folinic acid 'rescue'. This use is potentially lethal, and the timing and dose sizes of the folinic
acid MUST be very closely supervised by the prescribing doctor.

Timing of peak fall in blood count
Stomatitis maximal at 7–10 days, marrow suppression maximal at 2 weeks,
both can persist for 3–4 weeks.

Main unwanted effects
1. Gastrointestinal mucous membrane ulceration.
2. Nephrotoxic in high doses.
3. Rarely: alopecia, diarrhoea, (responds to codeine phosphate)
   rashes, lung and liver damage.
4. Intrathecal therapy may occasionally result in chemical arach-
   noiditis or leucoencephalopathy.

Practical points in administration
1. Extensively protein bound therefore displaced by salicylates,
   sulphonamides, warfarin.
2. The formulation as powder contains paroben preservatives
   therefore never use this for intrathecal use — always check that
   the vial is marked for i.t. use.
3. There will be increased toxicity when a dose is given when the
   patient has a 'fluid reservoir' e.g. ascites, pleural effusion.
4. With high dose i.v. use, if the drip 'tissues' and an appreciable
   amount of methotrexate is given into the subcutaneous tissues,
   prolong the folinic acid rescue for a further 24 hours.
5. Doses and timing of the folinic acid rescue vary according to the
   dose of methotrexate used but a typical use would be 120 mg of
   folinic acid in divided doses over 24 hours starting 18 hours after
   the methotrexate dose, followed by 15 mg orally every 6 hours
   for the following 48 hours.

PROCARBAZINE   Natulan

Routes of administration
Oral only: yellow capsules of 50 mg.

Main haematological uses
Hodgkin's disease, other lymphomas, second line treatment in myeloma.

Typical dose used
50–300 mg daily in divided doses in 4 or 6 weekly cycles.

Timing of peak fall in blood count
10 days to 2 weeks.

Main unwanted effects
1. Allergic skin reactions.
2. Anorexia, nausea and vomiting but these are usually only apparent for the first few days of any course and then resolve as the treatment continues.
3. Dose-limiting myelosuppression. Reversible.

Practical points in administration
1. Severe intolerance to alcohol — warn the patient.
2. Acts as a weak monoamine oxidase inhibitor therefore will potentiate narcotics, phenothiazines, alcohol, barbiturates. Hypertensive crises may occasionally be provoked by high tyramine-content foods.

6-THIOGUANINE   Lanvis

Routes of administration
Orally only: white tablets of 40 mg.
Rest of details as for 6-mercaptopurine except that the dose of thioguanine does not have to be adjusted when given simultaneously with allopurinol.

VINBLASTINE   Velbe

Routes of administration
i.v. only; made up with sterile water or saline.

Main haematological uses
Lymphomas. ALL if neuropathy has precluded further use of vincristine.

Typical dose used
10–20 mg stat dose once weekly or fortnightly.

Timing of peak fall in blood count
5–10 days. Recovery complete within 12–24 days of the injection.

Main unwanted effects
1. Reversible myelosuppression, particularly neutrophils.
2. Occasionally neurotoxic — as for vincristine, q.v.
3. Occasionally, vomiting, alopecia.

Practical points in administration
1. Vinblastine is as damaging as vincristine if extravasated so the same precautions must be observed.

VINCRISTINE   Oncovin

Routes of administration
i.v. only.

Main haematological uses
ALL, lymphomas.

Typical dose used
1.0–2.0 mg/m^2 (usually up to a maximum of 2.0 mg). Usually given weekly.

Timing of peak fall in blood count
Only rarely and then mildly myelosuppressive. Can be given relatively safely in the presence of marrow hypoplasia.

Main unwanted effects
1. Peripheral neuropathy common. First sympton commonly parasthusiae in fingers. Reduced/absent tendon reflexes seen in approximately 30% of patients. Rarely, isolated cranial nerve lesions. Autonomic neuropathy sometimes seen, e.g. colonic atony, vaso-vagal.
2. Alopecia in nearly half the patients. May persist for many weeks beyond the cessation of treatment but regrows eventually.
3. Abdominal cramps common. 30% become constipated. Paralytic ileus rare but well recognised.
4. Rarely: vomiting, diarrhoea, hepatotoxity.

Practical points in administration
1. Severe ulceration occurs with extravasation of the injection.
2. Warn the patient about the possibility of hair loss.
3. Give a prophylactic bulk laxative.
4. Never give vincristine intrathecally.
5. Take all complaints of persistent constipation seriously and bear in mind that paralytic ileus can occur.
6. Warn the patient who has experienced neuropathic side effects that they may last for many weeks after the treatment has stopped but that full recovery eventually is the norm.
7. Vincristine administration may result in a thrombocytosis and this is the basis for its use in benign conditions such as idiopathic thrombocytopenic purpura.

VINDESINE   Eldisine

Routes of administration
i.v. only.

Main haematological uses
ALL. Occasionally lymphoma.

Typical dose used
3 mg/m^2 weekly.

Timing of peak fall in blood count
3–5 days. Recovery in 7 days.

Main unwanted effects
1. Alopecia common.
2. Neurotoxicity as for vincristine but tends to be less severe and less progressive.
3. Dose limiting neutropenia.

Practical points in administration
1. Very damaging if extravasated. See general notes.
2. There is no cross resistance with vincristine.
3. Must never be given intrathecally.
4. The platelet count is usually unaffected and there may even be a thrombocytosis. Very rarely it can cause a drop in the platelet count.

REFERENCES

Carter S K 1980 Cancer chemotherapy — new developments and changing concepts. Drugs 20(5): 375–397
Clendeninn N J et al 1984 Cytotoxic drugs active in leukaemia. In: Goldman J M, Preisler H D (eds) Leukaemias. Butterworth, London
Davey P, Tudhope G R 1983 Anti-cancer chemotherapy. British Medical Journal 287: 110–113

24. TERMINAL CARE IN HAEMATOLOGICAL MALIGNANCY

With careful manipulation of drug therapy and practical procedures, a physically comfortable, pain-free death should virtually always be achievable. A mentally and emotionally comfortable death requires the combined efforts of the family, doctors, nurses and others. Detailed discussion of the psychosocial care of the dying patient is outside the scope of this book — a few, very brief points only are mentioned, but an extensive bibliography is given.

The decision to withdraw active treatment is frequently difficult to make. Most important is discussion with the patient about his/her future care, but it is also vital to talk with the family and everyone involved in the care of the patient, including nursing staff and the GP.

Do not assume that a seriously ill patient with a history of cancer is terminally ill. Benign reversible conditions may mimic advanced malignant disease.

The usual mode of death from advanced haematological disease is bone marrow failure i.e. haemorrhage and infection. Bone pain is common with myeloma, less frequent with leukaemia and lymphoma.

Try not to avoid the patient or relatives and friends. A dying patient is a constant reminder of our fallibility, and the challenge this makes to our confidence and self-esteem is all too frequently inadequately met by refusing to face up to it. Ideally *increase* the number of your visits to your patient. Physical contact and affection are important. Try not to shuffle about embarrassedly at the end of the bed. Sit down beside the patient and listen.

Find out from the patient who is most important to them. Unmarried or homosexual partners are all too frequently ignored by medical staff. Establish early on whether it is feasible and preferable for the patient to be looked after at home. Many families want this but may refuse if they are scared that they cannot cope. Efficient and fast liaison with the GP, social worker and district nurse will often effect the patient's discharge from hospital to an organised system of care at home. Start with a trial day or weekend at home. Give clear information about whom the family should contact when they are worried — 24 hour 'cover' must be arranged. Discuss the possibility of hospice care.

Encourage the relatives to feel needed — involve them in the day-to-day hospital care of the patient e.g. bedbaths, mealtimes.

Explain everything you are planning to them. Speak to the relatives by themselves but, very importantly, also talk with them about the illness together with the patient. Conspiracy between the doctors and the relatives to the exclusion of the patient is very seldom appropriate.

If possible, agree to all the special requirements of the dying patient. Arrange for special food, allow visits by small children, let them read all night if they want to. Necessary ward discipline will seldom be compromised by such actions. Positively tell the patient that you will try to arrange for anything that they want — often they will be too frightened of being thought a nuisance to ask.

Maintain good communication with all staff who will care for the patient — particularly the nursing staff. Also very important is the briefing of 'covering' housemen so that inappropriate investigations and treatment are not instigated. Write clear policy comments in the patient's notes.

Some dying patients may prefer the privacy and quiet of a single room. If this is not possible, ask the nursing staff if the screens can be drawn round the bed sometimes when friends and relatives visit. The death of a loved one is profoundly distressing at the best of times but can be made even worse if the last chance to be with them is witnessed by a ward full of people.

GENERAL PRACTICAL POINTS

1. Reduce TPR measurements to once daily — a reasonable compromise between 'being abandoned by the nurses' and 'not being left alone in peace'.
2. Always assume that apparently comatose patients can hear and understand you.
3. Explain to the patient why they have certain symptoms — it can be very reassuring that their doctor knows what is going on and is about to do something to try to relieve it.
4. Do not hesitate to ask for specialist help — e.g. from hospices about pain relief.
5. Intravenous cannulae:
   A permanent drip should be avoided if at all possible, but i.v. analgesics may occasionally be preferable to oral or i.m. Do not maintain infusion fluids — rapidly progressive renal failure is a relatively peaceful way in which to die and the encumbrance of the drip tubing is uncomfortable. A useful way of maintaining access to the circulation, if needed, is with a heparinised intermittent infusion 'butterfuly' needle, inserted well away from a joint and secured only with a gauze pad and a few pieces of non-allergic tape.
6. Limit investigations but do not abandon all of them, e.g. a chest X-ray is totally unnecessary in a chest infection that is not to be treated, but a judicious check of the haemoglobin may allow you to correct distressing symptoms due to anaemia.

7. Hypercalcaemia is always worth detecting and treating.
8. Symptom relief depends on careful clinical evaluation — a common fault is 'to leave them alone, they are dying' and this leads to inadequate palliation. For example, dyspnoea may be due to a pleural effusion, anaemia, chest infection, metabolic disturbance and appropriate treatment will render the patient much more comfortable.

THE MANAGEMENT OF SPECIFIC SYMPTOMS

Dry, sore mouth
1. Regular mouth toilet, at least b.d.
2. Prevent dehydration. Intravenous rehydration is seldom indicated. Sucking small pieces of ice will help (more comfortable if the ice is wrapped in a piece of gauze).
3. Dry mouth due to drugs (e.g. antihistamines, phenothiazines) or to anorexia (reduced stimulation to salivation): withdraw drugs if possible; give boiled sweets, chewing gum, artificial saliva.
4. Oral infection (usually candidiasis): treat with nystatin suspension (1 ml swilled around the mouth q.d.s.) and use it to paint the dentures. Prophylaxis is possible with amphotericin lozenges but they are rather unpalatable.
5. Aphthous ulceration and mucosal damage caused by cytotoxic drugs: try corticosteroid lozenges (e.g. Corlan 2.5 mg q.d.s.), chlorhexidine mouth wash or benzocaine anaesthetic 10 mg throat lozenges.

Pruritus and dry skin
Multifactorial and elusive pathogenesis.
1. Local measures: simple aqueous emollient creams are best. Avoid creams containing antibiotics. Creams containing camphor or menthol may have an anti-pruritic effect. Stop using soap. Calamine lotion may be helpful.
2. Systemic anti-pruritics: bile salt itch in obstructive jaundice may be seen in patients with lymphoma. It should respond to some degree to cholestyramine (1–2 sachets, p.o. 2–3 times daily) but this is an unpalatable drug. Oral anti-histamines can be tried although they are often not helpful.

Bed sores
1. Preventative: usual measures such as frequent turning, sheepskin undersheet and sheepskin 'wraps' for pressure areas, scrupulous drying of the skin after washing.
2. Treatment of established sores: probably no one method is better than another. Experienced nurses usually have their own favourite method, so follow local policy.

Dysphagia

1. Consider oesophageal candidiasis. Systemic anti-fungals are necessary to eradicate the infection but these are not indicated in the dying patient.
2. Pressure from mediastinal lymphadenopathy: dexamethasone 2–4 mg 6 hourly, and/or local radiotherapy.

Fever

Considerably adds to the debilitation. Treat symptomatically with tepid sponging, fan and anti-pyretics e.g. paracetamol or aspirin (caution in thrombocytopenic bleeding).

Anorexia

1. Correct any hypercalcaemia.
2. Small amount of brandy or sherry before meals.
3. Prednisolone 5–15 mg p.o. daily will stimulate appetitie.
4. Small portions of palatable food.

Anaemia

Progressive anaemia is a slow and distressing mode of death. Judicious use of packed cell transfusions, e.g. 2 units given via a butterfly needle, will make the patient more comfortable.

Urinary incontinence

This can be very distressing. Moving on and off bed-pans is also painful. Try penile tubing first in males but talk to the patient about the pros and cons of an indwelling catheter — many prefer to have one.

Vomiting

For suitable anti-emetic regimes see page 145.

Causes

1. Drugs e.g. opiates and cytotoxics.
2. Hypercalcaemia: for treatment see page 130.
3. Raised intracranial pressure: treat with dexamethasone 1–4 mg 6 hourly.

Bleeding

Thrombocytopenic bleeding is unpleasant and frightening. Give platelet transfusions where practical.

Constipation

Virtually always present in patients taking opiates, treat if symptomatic. The most practical treatment is the use of glycerin or Dulcolax suppositories given at a time to suit the patient. However, oral laxatives are sometimes necessary and a preparation that acts as both a stimulant and a faecal softener is usually best (e.g. Dioctyl syrup). Bisacodyl with lactulose is an alternative. Be wary of diarrhoea in patients taking opiates — it almost always represents 'overflow' around impacted faeces and manual extraction may be necessary.

Dyspnoea
Particular causes in haematological malignancy:
1. Cardiac failure secondary to anaemia.
2. Chest infection.
3. Mediastinal or cervical node obstruction (will usually respond to dexamethasone and/or local radiotherapy).
4. Opiates will suppress respiratory drive and are therefore excellent drugs to relieve the dyspnoea of the dying patient.
5. 'Death rattle' may be abolished by hyoscine hydrobromide 0.4 mg s.c. every 4 hours.
6. Oxygen therapy is not usually helpful, is uncomfortable and upsetting to the family.

Insomnia
1. Treat any underlying problem e.g. pain, dyspnoea, night sweats (may respond to indomethacin 50 mg nocte), anxiety.
2. Useful hypnotics: temazepam 10–20 mg nocte, dichloralphenazone 2 tabs nocte, chlormethiazole 2 caps nocte.

Depression and anxiety
1. This is obviously very common. The first approach is to listen and reassure — informal psychotherapy and support is often all that is needed.
2. Ideally, large oncology units will have access to a psychiatrist with expertise in the management of terminally ill patients.
3. Particularly useful drugs:
   Amitryptyline (has a sedative component) 25–100 mg nocte.
   Imipramine (less sedative) 20–100 mg daily in divided doses.
   Dothiepin 25–50 mg nocte.
4. Generally, small doses only are needed.
5. Tricyclic antidepressants and related compounds can take up to three weeks to have an effect.
6. Monoamine-oxidase inhibitors are too troublesome to use in this short-term situation and ECT is not indicated in the dying patient.
7. When anxiolytics are necessary, useful drugs are:
   a. Shorter acting: lorazepam 1 mg daily — 2 mg q.d.s.
   b. Longer acting: diazepam 2–10 mg t.d.s. or clobazam 10 mg once daily to q.d.s. or full dose at night only.

Pain relief
1. Assess the pain fully, i.e. how many sites are involved, what activities are limited, is sleep prevented, is the pain due to bone lesions, nerve compression (e.g. by malignant lymphadenopathy), visceral involvement (may be seen with lymphomas).
2. There is no place for 'p.r.n.' treatment in severe pain in terminal illness — treat pain prophylactically i.e. anticipate its recurrence rather than wait to treat it once it has returned.

3. If the pain is overwhelming start treatment with generous doses of opiates and then reduce the dose at leisure otherwise start with non-narcotic analgesics at a standard dose BUT review the situation at least once daily, ideally at each dose interval, until the pain is properly controlled.

4. Bone pain from advanced haematological malignancy will often respond to one or two doses of appropriate cytotoxic chemotherapy i.e. the tumour burden is temporarily diminished enough to abolish infiltrative pain.

5. Use appropriate adjunctive therapy, e.g. headache due to raised intracranial pressure will improve with dexamethasone. For the treatment of bone pain, add an anti-inflammatory agent to the analgesic regime.

6. 'Cocktails' of opiates with alcohol and syrup are not appropriate treatment. They are very sickly to take and some of their contents are unnecessary or even detrimental. Elixirs can be made up with just fruit juice.

7. Nocturnal pain may be prevented by giving a double dose of analgesic (plus a hypnotic) at bedtime. If this is ineffective, it is better to wake the patient to give them further doses rather than allow them to be woken by pain.

8. Parenteral analgesia is unnecessary except in exceptional circumstances, e.g. inability to swallow, sudden exacerbation of pain while stabilised on oral medication.

9. Keep analgesic regimes simple. Get used to a small number of effective drugs and become expert at manipulating their dosage. Increase the dose or move up to a stronger 'group' rather than give two or more different analgesics together or change to another preparation of similar potency. Beware of interactions e.g. do not mix a narcotic agonist-antagonist (e.g. pentazocine, buprenorphine) with narcotic agonists (e.g. codeine, morphine).

10. Avoid pethidine, pentazocine, dextromoramide and dipipanone as they are too short acting. Use methadone and levorphanol only with extreme caution as both tend to accumulate.

Specific analgesics

1. Non-narcotics:
   a. Aspirin: 300 mg tabs. Give 4-hourly. Sometimes large doses e.g. 1200 mg 4-hourly, may be necessary and are often well tolerated. Usually taken in soluble form, enteric-coated preparations may reduce dyspeptic side-effects.
   b. Paracetamol: 500 mg tabs. 2 tabs every 4–6 hours. Available as an elixir
   c. Naproxen: 250 mg dose, as capsules, tablets, elixir or suppository. Use 250–500 mg 8–12 hourly.

2. Weak narcotics:
   a. Codeine phophate tablets. Available as 15 mg, 30 mg, and 60 mg. Give 15–60 mg 4-hourly. Can use as syrup. Give prophylactic laxative. Codeine is approximately one tenth as potent as morphine, mg for mg
   b. Dihydrocodeine tartrate (DF 118). Give as tablets or syrup 30–60 mg, 4–6 hourly. Otherwise as for codeine.
3. Strong narcotics:
   a. Buprenorphine. Must be given sub-lingually and not just swallowed. Start at 0.2 mg 8 hourly but this can be increased, probably to a maximum of 1.2 mg 6-hourly (equivalent to approximately 50 mg of oral morphine sulphate 4-hourly). Occasional patients will not achieve analgesia for 6 hours, in which case half the six-hourly dose may be given every 3 hours. Do not give it with morphine. Side-effects include nausea, sweating, dizziness and sedation
   b. Morphine sulphate. The drug of choice for severe pain in terminal illness. The problems of addiction are non-existent in this group of patients and morphine can be used in high doses for long-term metastatic pain palliation without significant sedation. It is quite feasible for patients to lead a near-normal life (i.e. even at work) while taking doses of say, 300 mg daily

   It can be given as:
   (i)   Slow-release tablets: available as 10 mg, 30 mg, 60 mg, and 100 mg strengths. Give 12-hourly initially but it may be necessary to increase to 8-hourly
   (ii) Aqueous solution: 10 mg in 10 ml
   (iii) Suppository: 15 mg or 30 mg
   (iv) Parenteral bolus: i.v./i.m./s.c. diamorphine. Start diamorphine at ⅓ of the previous morphine dose (in mg)
   (v)   Subcutaneous infusion: this is simple and convenient way of providing even analgesia. It is especially useful in the ambulant patient. Dissolve the total 24 hour dose requirement in 10 ml of water and set the adjustable battery operated syringe driver to deliver this dose in 24 hours. The pump is connected to an anaesthetic extension set and the morphine is delivered via a 25 gauge butterfly needle inserted subcutaneously in the abdominal wall, and secured by non-allergic tape.

Start morphine at a dose of 10 mg (4-hourly except for the slow-release tablets) or 5 mg in small or elderly patients. Always give prophylactic laxatives and assess the need for prophylactic anti-emetics (latter seldom needed).

Start treatment with morphine as an in-patient   this is partly to allay the patients fears about the drug but also, more importantly, to be able to supervise the dose escalation closely and frequently.

Side-effects: confusion, drowsiness, vomiting (all usually only seen for the first few days of treatment) and constipation and nausea (may be long-term problems).

REFERENCES

Bonica J J 1982 Management of cancer pain. Acta Anaesthesiology of Scandinavia (Supplement) 26: 75–82
Kubler-Ross E 1969 On death and dying. Tavistock, London
Kuhse H, Hughes G 1982 Extraordinary means and the ethics of life. Journal of Medical Ethics 7: 74–82
Saunders C M (ed) 1978 The management of terminal disease. Edward Arnold, London
Twycross R G, Lack S A 1984 Therapeutics in terminal cancer. Pitman. London

Part 6
HAEMOSTASIS

25. HAEMOSTATIC FAILURE

DEFINITION

Inappropriate and excessive bleeding either spontaneous or in response to injury.

NORMAL HAEMOSTASIS

This depends on:
1. Local vascular constriction to decrease blood flow.
2. Platelet-vessel wall interaction with the formation of a haemostatic plug.
3. Interaction between soluble coagulation factors with the formation of a fibrin clot.
4. Appropriate fibrinolyic activity.

Although significant clinical bleeding can occur as a result of vascular abnormalities and abnormalities of fibrinolysis, the commonest and most important causes of bleeding are associated with disturbances of platelet plug and fibrin clot formation.

PRESENTATION

In disorders of haemostasis the bleeding manifestations are commonly at more than one site.
1. Acute bleeding:
   a. Spontaneous bruising or purpura
   b. Bleeding from mucous membranes, e.g. nose/mouth, gastrointestinal tract, urogenital tract, uterus post delivery
   c. Bleeding from venepuncture, intravenous cannulation and operation sites and from tooth sockets post dental extraction
   d. Bleeding into muscles, joints or deep tissues
   e. Cerebral haemorrhage.

2. Chronic bleeding:
   a. Epistaxes
   b. Skin bruising, either spontaneous or following trauma
   c. Purpura — commoner on dependent parts of body
   d. Menorrhagia.

AETIOLOGY

Platelet abnormalities

1. Quantitative
   a. Decreased bone marrow production:
      (i) Malignant marrow infiltration — leukaemia, myeloma, lymphoma
      (ii) Drugs — phenylbutazone, gold, co-trimoxazole, cytotoxics
      (iii) Severe megaloblastic anaemia
      (iv) Hypoplastic anaemia
   b. Decreased platelet survival:
      (i) Immune mechanisms:
          Primary — immune thrombocytopenia (ITP)
          Secondary — SLE, CLL, lymphoma, post transfusion
          Drugs — thiazides, quinine, quinidine, heparin, rifampicin, PAS, sulphonamides
      (ii) Excessive consumption:
          Disseminated intravascular coagulation (DIC)
          Thrombotic thrombocytopenic purpura (TTP)
          Sequestration with splenomegaly
          Cardiopulmonary bypass
          Dilution following massive, rapid blood transfusion.
2. Qualitative
   Platelet count variable from normal to modest decrease
   Prolonged bleeding time characteristic
   Abnormal in vitro platelet aggregation tests
   a. Inherited: e.g. Bernard Soulier syndrome, thrombasthenia and storage pool disease. These are rare
   b. Acquired: often show features of primary disease that causes platelet dysfunction e.g. myeloproliferative diseases, uraemia, paraproteinaemias
      Drugs an important cause, e.g. aspirin and non-steroidal anti-inflammatory drugs.

Coagulation factor deficiencies

Congenital
Usually single factor deficiencies. Sometimes clinically apparent at birth, but mild deficiencies may not become apparent until adolescence or adult life, e.g. Haemophilia A (Factor VIII) and B (Factor IX, Christmas disease) (p. 189), von Willebrand's disease (p. 200), Factor XI deficiency. Other deficiencies are rare.

Acquired
Commoner.
Usually associated with multiple factor deficiencies, secondary to underlying disease or drug treatment.

1. Decreased production: e.g. liver disease, Vitamin K deficiency — neonates (especially premature), malabsorption, obstructive jaundice.
2. Increased consumption: disseminated intravascular coagulation (DIC).
3. Circulating inhibitors:
   e.g. antibodies — especially to Factor VIII (5-10% of severe haemophiliacs, pregnancy, associated with autoimmune disease, idiopathic, especially elderly) and associated with SLE.
4. Drugs: heparin and warfarin.
5. Dilution: massive, rapid blood transfusion.

POINTS TO NOTE IN HISTORY

1. Sex: 85% of congenital factor deficiencies occur in males.
2. Bleeding: immediate or prolonged following cuts suggests thrombocytopenia or platelet dysfunction. Delayed bleeding suggests coagulation factor deficiency.
3. Family history: may indicate congenital factor deficiency.
4. Previous bleeding episodes: especially associated with trauma, operations or dental extractions. May indicate a congenital bleeding disorder.
5. Drugs: especially anticoagulants, aspirin, non-steroidal anti-inflammatory agents and cytotoxics.
6. Past medical history: especially of liver disease, renal failure and bone marrow dysfunction (e.g. hypoplasia, leukaemia).
7. Uterine bleeding: previous menorrhagia or severe previous post natal bleeding.
8. Clinical situation: e.g. neonate, obstructive jaundice, recent massive blood transfusion or conditions associated with DIC.

POINTS TO NOTE ON EXAMINATION

1. Skin bruising or purpura and mucosal bleeding: widespread bruising suggests coagulation factor deficiency while purpura or mucosal bleeding suggests platelet bleeding.
2. Muscle or joint bleeding: suggests congenital coagulation factor deficiency.
3. Multisite bleeding: suggests haemostatic failure, while localised bleeding requires the elimination of a medical or surgical cause.
4. Oral petechiae or fundal haemorrhage: a sign of serious haemostatic failure. Can precede a cerebral haemorrhage, especially in the presence of thrombocytopenia.
5. Look for clinical signs of liver disease and check for splenomegaly.

LABORATORY ASSESSMENT

There is no substitute for an accurate laboratory assessment *before* treatment is started:

1. Obtain samples from a fresh venepuncture and *not* from an indwelling i.v. cannula
2. Citrate should be the anticoagulant used. Sample bottles can usually be obtained from the laboratory. *Do not* use ESR bottles
3. Send the samples to the laboratory with the minimum of delay.

Test available

1. Blood count, blood film and platelet count: there may be abnormalities of red cells and white cells suggesting leukaemia, hypoplasia or DIC, as well as the platelet count itself.
2. Prothrombin time (PT): indicates extrinsic pathway activity. Usually reported as a prothrombin ratio (PTR) or British Ratio (BR) of the patient's PT to that of a normal control plasma.
3. Activated partial thromboplastin time with kaolin (APTT): intrinsic pathway activity. Varieties of this test include KCCT and PTTK. Time (in seconds) reported along with the APTT of a normal plasma. Can also be carried out with a 50:50 mixture of patient and normal plasma, both tested immediately and after 1 hours 37°C incubation. Correction of a prolonged time indicates coagulation factor deficiency while lack of correction indicates the presence of an inhibitor.
4. Thrombin time (TT): measures the thrombin-fibrinogen reaction. Is prolonged with either fibrinogen deficiency or interference with the reaction (e.g. heparin or FDPs). In the presence of heparin, a *reptilase time* is normal while the TT is prolonged.

5. Fibrinogen level.
6. Fibrin(ogen) degradation products (FDPs): reflects fibrinolytic activity. Most commonly raised following blood transfusion and post operatively. Very raised levels are often indicative of DIC. Requires special sample bottle, usually obtained from the laboratory.
7. Fibrin monomers (FMs): presence indicates excessive thrombin activity. Often found in active DIC.
8. Bleeding time (BT): using a standard spring loaded template device. Prolonged with thrombocytopenia, platelet dysfunction and in von Willebrand's disease.
9. In vitro platelet aggregation: for assessing potential platelet dysfunction.
10. Coagulation factor assays: for accurate diagnosis of factor deficiencies. Most commonly required are Factor VIII, Factor IX and Factor XI.
11. Euglobulin lysis time (ELT): overall test indicating fibrinolytic activity. Result usually reported with that for a normal plasma control.

NB: Generally the *whole blood clotting time* is no longer used as it is too imprecise. The *thrombotest* is for controlling oral anticoagulant therapy and is not a coagulation screening test.

Suggested tests for acute bleeding

1. Minimum screen: blood count and platelet count, PT and APTT (if APTT is prolonged then repeat on a mixture of patient and normal plasma).
2. If available: TT, FDPs and FMs and fibrinogen level. It is always worthwhile to freeze some citrated plasma in case further more complex tests are required.

Suggested tests for longstanding bleeding disorder

As above, but in addition the following tests can be done where appropriate:

1. Bleeding time.
2. In vitro platelet aggregation.
3. Euglobulin lysis time.
4. Specific factor assays.

INTERPRETATION OF BASIC SCREENING TESTS

1. Decreased platelets with normal coagulation (see Ch. 11). Associated anaemia and granulocytopenia suggests hypoplasia. Circulating blasts suggests leukaemia.
   Consider an urgent bone marrow which may confirm the diagnosis of hypoplasia, leukaemia or marrow infiltration, or suggest decreased platelet production. A normal marrow suggests peripheral platelet destruction, consumption or loss from the circulation.

2. Normal platelet count with abnormal coagulation
   a. Prolonged PT, normal APTT:
      (i)   Warfarin or related anticoagulants
      (ii) Liver disease
      (iii) Factor VII deficiency (rare)
   b. Normal PT, prolonged APTT:
      (i)   Deficiencies of factors XII, XI, IX or VIII. With factor XII deficiency there is no bleeding disorder. Haemophilia and Christmas disease are almost always found in males. Factor XI deficiency is commoner in Jews. Von Willebrand's disease (p. 200) may be associated with a prolonged APPT
   c. Prolonged PT, prolonged APTT:
      As isolated deficiencies in the final common pathway are rare, this usually indicates multiple (and therefore acquired) factor deficiencies, e.g. liver disease, DIC, massive rapid banked blood transfusion, Vitamin K deficiency.
3. Decreased platelets with abnormal coagulation:
   a. Massive rapid stored blood transfusion
   b. Liver disease (thrombocytopenia usually secondary to splenomegaly)
   c. DIC.

MANAGEMENT

General
1. It is important to establish the nature and severity of the haemostatic defect both clinically and by laboratory testing in order that appropriate treatment may be given.
2. Repeat testing following treatment, particularly if surgical intervention is contemplated, should be done.
3. If bleeding continues following *adequate* replacement therapy a local cause for bleeding should be considered.

Thrombocytopenia
Spontaneous bleeding usually only occurs when platelet count is $< 20 \times 10^9/1$, though if there is associated platelet dysfunction (e.g. leukaemia or myeloproliferative disease) or infection, bleeding may occur at higher platelet counts. If count is $< 20 \times 10^9/1$ or there is bleeding, give ABO compatible platelets 1 unit/10 kg body weight. This may need to be repeated every 24–48 hours or more often if blood loss is continuing. Regular platelet counts should be performed. More units are required if there is associated infection. Giving platelets to patients with immune based thrombocytopenia is seldom successful as the platelets are rapidly destroyed following infusion. However intra-operative platelet transfusion may be given during surgical procedures in these patients.

Coagulation factor deficiency

   1. *Fresh frozen plasma (FFP)*
      Contains all coagulation factors (though has decreased amounts of factors V and VIII) but no platelets. Not to be confused with PPF (plasma protein fraction) — that contains only albumin and electrolyte. It is the treatment of choice for most factor deficiencies except haemophilia and Christmas disease. Give either ABO specific or group AB FFP. Give initially 2–4 units depending on the degree of coagulation abnormality.

      It is advisable, where possible, to repeat the coagulation screen following treatment and to give further FFP if the screen remains abnormal and bleeding continues. Beware of fluid overload, especially in infants, the elderly and those with chronic liver disease.

   2. Cryoprecipitate and specific factor concentrates: Mainly used in the management of haemophilia A and B. Cryoprecipitate contains factor VIII and is a useful source of fibrinogen. Freeze dried concentrates of factor VIII and factor IX are available. The latter also contains factors II and X but is not often used therapeutically for deficiencies of these factors. For further information see Chapter 28 on haemophilia and Chapter 29 on blood component therapy.

   3. Vitamin K: useful in vitamin K deficiency, liver disease and warfarin reversal (p. 185). For adults give 10 mg p.o. or slow i.v. daily (not i.m. as severe local bruising can result).

NB: Fresh blood contains relatively small amounts of platelets and coagulation factors, and is not recommended as a substitute for platelet concentrate or FFP.

MANAGEMENT OF SPECIFIC CONDITIONS

Disseminated intravascular coagulation

This is caused by the release into the circulation of a procoagulant, activating the coagulation pathway in vivo. This results in:

   1. Consumption of coagulation factors and platelets resulting in bleeding.
   2. Thrombi in the microcirculation with resulting organ damage.

Causes

   1. Acute severe infections, especially Gram negative septicaemia.
   2. Obstetric emergencies, e.g. abruptio placentae, amniotic fluid embolism, retained dead fetus, severe pre-eclampsia.
   3. Incompatible blood transfusion.
   4. After major surgery.
   5. Severe trauma or burns.
   6. Severe shock, hypoxia or acidosis.
   7. Malignancy: e.g. promyelocytic leukaemia and mucin-secreting adenocarcinoma.

Diagnosis

Laboratory tests in acute DIC may show:
1. Prolonged PT, APTT, TT and reduced fibrinogen.
2. Thrombocytopenia.
3. Raised FDPs.
4. Fragmented cells on the blood film.

Treatment
1. Most important is the vigorous treatment of the underlying condition (see above).
2. If bleeding is prominent treat with FFP and platelet concentrate as appropriate.
3. Cryoprecipitate can be useful as the levels of factor VIII and fibrinogen may be low in DIC.
4. Heparin is *not* of proven value in DIC and the use of anti-fibrinolytic drugs is contraindicated.

Liver disease

Bleeding is usually from local sites (e.g. varices, peptic ulcer) exacerbated by associated coagulation abnormalities. Acute liver failure can be associated with DIC.

Specific therapy is usually required for:
1. Severe bleeding associated with abnormal coagulation tests. Give 2–4 units of FFP and then repeat the coagulation screen. If still abnormal and bleeding continues give further FFP. Start vitamin K 10 mg slow i.v. daily.
2. Before surgery or liver biopsy. If not urgent give vitamin K 10mg p.o. daily for five days and repeat the PT. If ratio is < 1.3 surgery or biopsy can go ahead. If correction is not successful, or surgery is urgently required use FFP. Recheck the coagulation screen post infusion and prior to any biopsy or surgical procedure, giving further FFP as necessary. Careful monitoring after surgical procedures is necessary and further FFP may need to be given.

If FFP is ineffective, or there is danger of fluid overload, factor IX concentrates can be given. These can precipitate DIC and are thrombogenic and should only be given after consultation with the haematologist.

Patients with liver disease may be thrombocytopenic. If surgery or biopsy is essential give platelet concentrate (p. 207).

Dilution

Associated with the rapid administration of large amounts of stored blood which is deficient in platelets and coagulation factors. Give one unit of FFP for every five to six units of stored blood if given at a rate faster than two units/hour. Platelet concentrate may be required if the platelet count falls to $< 70 \times 10^9/1$. Monitor coagulation screen and give further therapy as necessary.

NB: If coagulation screen is normal, and platelet count $> 70 \times 10^9/1$ then a local cause for bleeding should be sought.

Anticoagulants

See Chapter 27.

Cardiopulmonary bypass

Postoperative bleeding in these patients may be caused by:

1. Thrombocytopenia. Due to trapping of platelets in the extracorporeal circuit. Give platelet concentrate.
2. Heparin effect. Can be shown by a prolonged TT with normal reptilase time. Protamine sulphate may be required.
3. Dilutional coagulopathy due to transfusion of large amounts of stored blood (see above).

REFERENCES

Ingram G I C, Brozovic M, Slater N G P 1982 Bleeding disorders: investigation and management, 2nd end. Blackwell, Oxford
Ockelford P A, Carter C J 1982 DIC: The application and utility of diagnostic tests. Seminars in thrombosis and haemostasis 8(3): 192–216

26. THROMBOSIS

PATHOGENESIS

1. Stasis, particularly in venous thrombosis.
2. Endothelial damage, particularly in arterial thrombosis.
3. Changes in blood constituents, 'hypercoagulability':
   a. Changes in coagulation with excess, inappropriate thrombin generation
   b. Changes in platelet behaviour
   c. Changes in blood viscosity (raised haematocrit).

CLINICAL ASSESSMENT OF RISK FACTORS

Venous thrombosis

The following predisposing factors should be considered in the selection of preoperative patients for low-dose heparin prophylaxis:

1. Increasing age (especially > 40 years).
2. Obesity (> 10% above mean body weight for age, height and sex).
3. Immobility e.g. post CVA or MI, especially those with CCF.
4. Previous history of DVT.
5. Varicose veins.
6. Cancer.
7. Major abdominal, gynaecological and hip operations.
8. Trauma to lower limb, especially fractured neck of femur.
9. Contraceptive pill or oestrogen therapy.
10. Pregnancy and puerperium.
11. Polycythaemia.
12. Family history of venous thrombosis.

Arterial thrombosis

The following are risk factors for arterial thrombosis and can be used as a guide to selection of patients for both primary and secondary prevention of coronary artery disease.

1. Cigarette smoking.
2. Hypertension.
3. Genetic factors (e.g. first degree relative with history of premature coronary artery disease).
4. Hyperlipidaemia.
5. Gout.
6. Diabetes mellitus.
7. Polycythaemia.

Currently the best predictor of the risk of reinfarction following an MI, and thus a guide to a potentially treatable 'high risk' group, is an abnormal ECG treadmill exercise test one month post infarction.

Investigation of suspected 'hypercoagulability'

Just as low clotting factors can lead to a bleeding tendency, it is suggested that increased coagulability of the blood may lead to thrombosis.

Laboratory tests for hypercoagulability may be useful in the following situations:

1. To define 'at risk' groups e.g. preoperatively or post MI.
2. Venous thrombosis with no clear disposing cause, especially in the young patient.
3. Venous thrombosis in more than one member of a family.
4. Recurrent venous thrombosis and/or pulmonary embolism.
5. Retinal vein occlusion.

The following tests when available may demonstrate a hypercoagulable state but are of less predictive value than the clinical risk factors above; many are only available in specialist centres.

1. Tests to detect increased thrombin activation:
   a. Shortened activated partial thromboplastin time (APTT)
   b. Screening test for fibrin monomers
   c. Fibrinopeptide A
   d. Detection of high MWt soluble complexes of fibrin monomer
   e. Increased ratio of F VIII RAG to F VIII C.
2. Tests to detect increased platelet activity:
   a. Platelet count to exclude thrombocytosis.
   b. Spontaneous platelet aggregation — visual technique
   c. In vitro platelet aggregation techniques.
   d. Platelet factor 4 and ß thromboglobulin levels.

3. Tests of fibrinolysis:
   a. FDPs (can be increased as a result of excess fibrin breakdown)
   b. Euglobulin clot lysis time (ELT) pre and post venous occlusion at 80mm Hg. This tests fibrinolytic activity and capacity (the post occlusion time should be significantly reduced). Decreased fibrinolysis can be associated with an increased risk of venous thrombosis.
4. Tests measuring natural inhibitors of coagulation:
   a. Anti-thrombin III — a decrease is associated with increased risk of venous thrombosis.
5. Tests related to blood viscosity:
   a. Haemoglobin and PCV
   b. Whole blood viscosity.

DIAGNOSIS OF SUSPECTED THROMBOEMBOLISM

Deep Venous thrombosis (DVT)

Clinical signs

1. Calf DVT; commonest signs are:
   a. Calf muscle induration present in 68% of patients.
   b. Minimal unilateral oedema 52%
   c. Local increased temperature 34%
   d. Calf tenderness 25%.
   NB: Only 50% of patients with demonstrable DVT have clinical signs. 20% of patients with clinical signs *do not* have DVTs
2. DVT above the knee; clinical signs are more reliable:
   a. Pain and tenderness over veins in thigh or calf
   b. Swelling of leg (can be extensive and decrease arterial circulation)
   c. Superficial veins dilated.

Venography

1. Most accurate.
2. Can visualise the exact site, extent and nature of the thrombus including external and common iliac veins.
3. Invasive, and can be painful (premedication with 10–20 mg of Omnopon is recommended).
4. Can cause post venography DVT (< 3%).
5. Minimal danger of precipitating a PE.

^{125}I fibrinogen uptake test

1. Radioactive fibrinogen is injected i.v. and is taken up into an *active* thrombus and can be detected as a 'hot spot'.
2. Accurate for calf vein thrombi, but less accurate in upper third of thigh and cannot detect thrombi in pelvic veins.

3. Invasive, and need to prevent radioactive iodine uptake by thyroid by concurrent administration of potassium iodide.
4. False positives with haematoma, gross oedema, inflammatory reactions, incisions and arthritis. Care needs to be taken with interpretation in superficial thrombophlebitis and varicose veins.
5. Contraindicated in pregnancy and lactation.

Impedance plethysmography
1. Changes in calf blood volume following the inflation and subsequent release of pressure cuff round the thigh are measured. DVT results in a reduction of the maximum venous volume of the calf and a decrease in the rate of venous outflow.
2. Accurate in detecting proximal vein thrombi.
3. Non-invasive.
4. Will not detect most calf vein thrombi and small non-occlusive proximal thrombi may be missed.
5. Widely used in North America in combination with ^{125}I fibrinogen uptake as an alternative to venography.

Ultrasound
1. In a patent vein the velocity of venous flow can be briefly increased by compressing the extremity and this can be detected by the ultrasound probe. In the presence of venous occlusion such augmented signals are decreased or absent.
2. Fairly accurate in detecting occlusive proximal thrombi.
3. Simple, rapid and non-invasive.
4. Less accurate in detecting non-occlusive proximal thrombi and calf vein thrombi.

Thermography
1. Uses an infra-red camera to detect the increased temperature in a limb overlying an area of active thrombosis.
2. Most accurate for calf vein thrombi.
3. False positives with cellulitis, inflammation, haematoma and superficial thrombophlebitis.

Pulmonary embolus

Clinical (commonest findings)
1. Pulmonary infarction:
   a. Dyspnoea and tachypnoea
   b. Pleuritic pain and haemoptysis.
2. Acute cor pulmonale:
   a. Dyspnoea and tachypnoea
   b. Apprehension and syncope
   c. Sweating and cyanosis
   d. Gallop rhythm and increased pulmonary second sound.

Chest X-ray
1. Can be valuable but normal in 25% of cases.
2. Commonest findings are linear or wedge shaped opacities, small pleural effusions, and (in massive emboli) areas of oligo-and hyperaemia.

ECG
1. Abnormalities are present in most patients with large emboli.
2. Not specific (only 10% show S1-Q3-T3 pattern).
3. Useful in excluding acute MI.

Arterial oxygen saturation
1. Difficult to interpret in patients with pre-existing cardiopulmonary disease.
2. The decrease in oxygen saturation reflects the extent of the embolic process.

Perfusion lung scanning
1. Virtually non-invasive.
2. False positives with pneumonia, pleural effusion and chronic obstructive airways disease.
3. False negatives possible with large proximal emboli.
4. Diagnostic specificity increased by:
   a. typical lesions on scan
   b. Accompanying CXR — an abnormality in the scan is more likely to be due to embolus than other pulmonary disease if CXR is normal
   c. Accompanying ventilation scan — typically in PE abnormality on perfusion scan not reflected on ventilation scan.

Pulmonary angiography
1. Accurate.
2. Invasive.
3. Usually only available in specialist centres.
4. Necessary if embolectomy is being considered.

Assessment of deep veins
1. PE almost always associated with DVT.
2. With suspected PE but no access to either lung scanning or angiography the presence of a DVT supports a diagnosis of PE.
3. Best to use venography, if available.

REFERENCES

Davies J A, McNicol G P 1978 Blood coagulation in pathological thrombus formation and the detection in blood of a thrombotic tendency. British Medical Bulletin 34(2): 113–121
Morris G K, Mitchell J R A 1978 Clinical management of venous thrombo-embolism. British Medical Bulletin 34(2): 169–175
Prentice C R M (ed) 1981 Thrombosis. Clinics in Haematology 10(2)

27. ANTICOAGULANT, THROMBOLYTIC AND ANTI-PLATELET THERAPY

These agents can be used:
1. To prevent initial thrombotic events — *primary prophylaxis* e.g. low dose heparin in the prevention of postoperative deep vein thrombosis (DVT) and pulmonary embolus (PE).
2. In the treatment of established thrombosis — *therapeutic* e.g. use of i.v. heparin and oral warfarin in the treatment of established DVT.
3. To prevent further thrombosis or embolism following an initial thrombotic event — *secondary prophylaxis*, e.g. anti-platelet agents or warfarin following myocardial infarction.

INDIVIDUAL DRUGS AND THEIR CLINICAL USE

Heparin

Low dose, short term

Indication
Prevention of DVT and PE postoperatively and post myocardial infarction.

Dosage
5000 units calcium heparin s.c. with the premedication — then 12 hourly until patient ambulant.

Control
None required.

Complications
Minor bleeding (e.g. wound haematomata) in a minority of patients.

Special precautions
Haemorrhagic conditions; concurrent administration of aspirin and related drugs.

Low dose, long term

Indication
Treatment of DVT in pregnancy instead of warfarin during first trimester (risk of fetal malformation) and from 37 weeks (more risk of haemorrhage with warfarin).

Dosage
5000 units s.c. b.d. for calf vein thrombi.
Adjusted dose for proximal thrombi.

Control
Only necessary in patients with proximal thrombi. Aim for heparin level of 0.1 to 0.3 units/ml.

Complications
Minor bleeding; osteoporosis (rare and associated with prolonged administration).

Full dose

Indication
Established DVT or PE.

Dosage
Very variable; average 25,000 to 40,000 units daily.

Administration
Continuous i.v. infusion preferable to intermittent injection. Use syringe pump; electronic drop counter (IVAC); paediatric burette; i.v. infusion in saline.

Control
Daily APPT. Aim at time 2–3 times the control (70–100 sec).

Duration of treatment
Calf DVTs: 3 days. Start warfarin on day 1.
Proximal DVTs and pulmonary emboli: 7–10 days. Start warfarin on either day 5 or 8.

Complications
Bleeding; immune thrombocytopenia (rare).

Treatment of overdosage
Stop infusion. Usually sufficient as heparin is rapidly cleared from circulation (half life one hour). If urgent reversal required give 50 mg protamine sulphate i.v. over 5 minutes.

Special precautions
See under **low dose, short term** above.

Warfarin

Indications
1. Established DVT or PE.
2. Mitral valve disease, especially if accompanied by atrial fibrillation.
3. Post heart valve replacement.
4. Following transient cerebral ischaemic episodes (TIA). Does carry a risk of cerebral haemorrhage especially if continued for more than one year (also see anti-platelet drugs).
5. Following myocardial infarction (MI). Benefit remains uncertain.

Dosage

If following heparin, start warfarin three days before heparin withdrawal.

Avoid large single loading doses (can cause severe bleeding).

Give warfarin for three days and check a prothrombin time (PT) on the fourth day having stopped any heparin 12 hours previously.

Normal sized adult — 10; 10; 5 mg

Small adult and elderly — 10; 5; 5 mg

Adjust dose of warfarin until PT is in therapeutic range (see below).

Control

PT as expressed as a ratio to a normal control plasma, or thrombotest.

Therapeutic range

Prothrombin time ratio 2–4.

Thrombotest 6–15%.

Duration of treatment

1. Calf vein DVT: three months.
2. Proximal DVT: minimum six months.
3. Small PE: minimum six months.
4. Extensive proximal DVT or large PE: at least one year.
5. Recurrent DVT or PE: long term.
6. Heart valve disease or replacement: long term.
7. TIA: six months to one year.
8. MI: up to two years.

Withdrawal of treatment

Gradually over two weeks (though there is conflicting evidence over 'rebound' hypercoagulability following sudden withdrawal).

Complications

1. Bleeding. Can be enhanced by concurrent administration of certain drugs (see appendix).
2. Rarely alopecia, rash, diarrhoea and 'purple toes' syndrome.

Treatment of overdosage

1. Ratio 5–8 or thrombotest < 5% but no bleeding. Stop warfarin for 24–48 hours. Reintroduce drug at lower dosage and retest in 2–7 days.
2. Ratio 5–8 or thrombotest < 5% and minor bleeding, or BCR over 8 without bleeding. Stop warfarin for 48 hours and retest on third day before restarting warfarin at lower dose.
3. Ratio > 5 or thrombotest < 5% and serious bleeding.

Stop drug. Give either vitamin K, 5–10 mg i.v. (or more if warfarin is not to be reintroduced) or two units fresh frozen plasma (FFP). Repeat as necessary. Reintroduce warfarin at lower dose when appropriate.

NB: Vitamin K can interfere with subsequent control for several weeks, and can take 12–24 hours to have a corrective effect.

For urgent reversal of warfarin activity e.g. for emergency surgery, stop drug and give at least 2 units of FFP. Repeat at 12 and 24 hours if necessary.

Absolute contraindications
1. Haemorrhagic diathesis.
2. Severe hypertension.
3. Previous cerebral haemorrhage.
4. CNS trauma.
5. Gastrointestinal bleeding.

NB: Breast feeding is no longer considered a contraindication, especially if the baby has received vitamin K.

Relative contraindications
1. Uraemia.
2. Liver disease.
3. Chronic alcoholism.
4. Subacute bacterial endocarditis.

Thrombolytic drugs

Streptokinase (SK) and urokinase (UK)

Indications
1. Massive proximal DVT.
2. Massive and submassive PE.
3. Sometimes in arterial thrombosis.

Dosage
1. SK — loading dose of 250 000 units over 30 minutes i.v. followed by 100 000 units hourly for 48–96 hours.
2. UK — loading dose of 4400 units/kg i.v. over 10 minutes, then 4400 units hourly for 12–24 hours.

Both drugs should be followed by conventional dose of heparin and warfarin.

Control
Thrombin time should be regularly checked and kept 2 to 4 times a normal control.

Complications
1. Bleeding with both SK and UK.
2. Allergic and febrile reactions with SK (can be ameliorated by adding hydrocortisone to the infusion).

Treatment of overdosage
Stop the drug. Usually all that is necessary as both rapidly cleared from circulation.

With serious bleeding can give an anti-fibrinolytic (e.g. tranexamic acid 500 mg i.v.) and if necessary FFP.

Absolute contraindications
1. Recent (< 2 months) CVA.
2. Active internal bleeding.

Relative contraindications
1. Recent arterial punctures.
2. Severe hypertension (> 200mm Hg systolic, > 110mm Hg diastolic).
3. Pregnancy.
4. Recent operation (< 10 days).

NB: Although there are now well defined clinical situations where the use of SK or UK is indicated they should both be used with great caution. It is fair to say that they should only be used:
1. By someone experienced in their use.
2. In centres where facilities exist for both venography and pulmonary angiography, and where adequate monitoring can be accomplished.

The greatest care should be exercised in recent postoperative patients and those in whom there has been a recent arterial puncture.

It should also be noted that the dosages given are only general guidelines, and the manufacturers instructions should always be consulted prior to administration.

Anti-platelet drugs

Indications
1. Post myocardial infarction.
2. Transient cerebral ischaemia.
3. Prosthetic heart valve replacement.
4. Digital ischaemia associated with thrombocytosis.

Drug and dosage
1. Myocardial infarction: either aspirin, 300 mg daily, or sulphinpyrazone, 200 mgs t.d.s., started within one month of infarction and continued for at least one and up to two years.
2. TIA: aspirin (either low dose, 300 mgs daily, or high dose, 300 mgs q.d.s.), long term.
3. Prosthetic heart valve replacement: use in combination with warfarin anticoagulation. Either dipyridamole, 100 mg q.d.s. or low dose aspirin, 300 mg daily, long term.
4. Digital ischaemia associated with thrombocytosis: aspirin 300 mg q.d.s.

Control
Not required.

Complications
Aspirin prolongs the bleeding time, while sulphinpyrazone and dipyridamole do not. Aspirin in combination with an oral anticoagulant can lead to an increased incidence of bleeding.

Special precautions

History of peptic ulceration; hepatic disease (sulphinpyrazone); anticoagulant administration (especially aspirin).

NB: The indications, drugs and dosages represented here are based on a large number of recent clinical trials and should be taken as general guidelines only.

APPENDIX

Drug interactions with warfarin

Drugs which increase the anticoagulant effect of warfarin

Alcohol — when taken in occasional excess ('binge').

Antibiotics (penicillin, sulphonamides, tetracyclines, cephalosporins).

Anti-inflammatory analgesics (aspirin, indomethacin, phenylbutazone).

Oral hypoglycaemics (tolbutamide, chlorpropamide, phenformin).

Anti-depressants (tricyclics, phenothiazines).

Laxatives.

Thyroxine and antithyroid drugs.

Allopurinol.

Drugs which decrease the anticoagulant effect of warfarin

Barbiturates.

Phenytoin.

Alcohol — with *regular* drinkers.

Rifampicin.

Cimetidine.

Diuretics — occasionally, especially spironolactone.

REFERENCES

Bell W R, Meek A G 1979 Guidelines for the use of thrombolytic agents. New England Journal of Medicine 301(23): 1266–1270

Buckler P, Douglas A S 1983 Anti-thrombotic treatment. British Medical Journal 287: 196–198

Mackie M J, Douglas A S 1978 Oral anticoagulants in arterial disease. British Medical Bulletin 34(2): 177–182

Webster J 1983 Anti-platelet drugs. British Journal of Hospital Medicine 30(1): 45–50

28. HAEMOPHILIA AND VON WILLEBRAND'S DISEASE

HAEMOPHILIA

Definition

A bleeding disorder caused by an inherited deficiency of clotting factor VIII (Haemophilia A) or IX (Haemophilia B or Christmas Disease). Haemophilia A and B are clinically indistinguishable and of similar severity, though A is more common.

Inheritance

Haemophilia A and B are both sex linked disorders, and hence affect almost exclusively males. Female carriers have on average a level of factor VIII or IX 50% of normal, but variation is wide and some carriers may exhibit a bleeding tendency for instance during surgery. Homozygous female haemophiliacs are extremely rare (occurring when the father is a haemophiliac and the mother a carrier). Spontaneous mutation is common, about 30% of haemophiliacs having no family history of the disorder.

Severity

Clinical severity is related to factor levels measured in clotting assays (normal 50–150 i.u./ml) = 50–150%.

Factor levels	Clinical severity	Type of bleeding
> 5%	Mild	On trauma only
2-5%	Moderate	Variable — severe problems with trauma; some spontaneous bleeding but infrequent in most patients
< 2%	Severe	Frequent spontaneous bleeds in most patients

Clinical disability does vary considerably between haemophiliacs with similar factor levels, and even at different times in the life of one individual. Physical and even emotional stress may be associated with increasing frequency of bleeds, but in general the bleeding events tend to be less frequent in adults than in children.

189

CLINICAL FEATURES

Age at presentation

Most haemophiliacs are clinically normal at birth and the bleeding tendency then presents usually between six months and two years, though sometimes, especially in mild cases, much later. Occasionally there is abnormal bleeding at or around birth, e.g. cerebral haemorrhage, bleeding from umbilical cord or after circumcision. The defect is demonstrable on clotting assays at birth and even in the foetus in utero, and so the diagnosis can be established at this time, but most clinical problems tend to appear when the child begins to move around independently.

Types of bleeding

Joints

Major site of apparently spontaneous bleeding. Knees, ankles, elbows, hips and shoulders are most common. The earliest manifestation is pain, followed by warmth, swelling and immobility of joint. Fluid may be demonstrated within the joint space. It must be stressed strongly that the patient is in general the best judge of the presence and severity of joint bleeds, and that absence of clinical signs does not negate the diagnosis. Chronic joint bleeds lead to persistent swelling, effusions, loss of movement and eventually ankylosis of the joint. Damaged joints may show a spiralling tendency to bleed more often (so called 'target joint') and chronic arthritis may be an additional source of pain. Ankylosed joints however tend to be painless and free from bleeds.

Soft tissue bleeding

Muscle and other soft tissue bleeds are common and may be accompanied by extensive surface ecchymoses. They are usually associated with some degree of trauma, though this may be slight. They often require more treatment for full resolution than a joint bleed of similar clinical severity. Serious complications are relatively common, in particular nerve and vascular compression. Bleeds in the hand must always be treated very actively and other relatively common problem sites are the ilio-psoas and gluteal areas. Ilio-psoas bleeds may present with abdominal pain (if right-sided they may mimic appendicitis) and signs of femoral nerve compression are often present.

Generalised bruising is surprisingly often absent, though many newly diagnosed haemophiliac children do present with a possible diagnosis of 'battered baby syndrome'.

CNS bleeding

Surprisingly uncommon but if intracerebral usually has devastating results — death or severe hemiplegia. Subdural or extradural haematoma may also occur and have a relatively good prognosis if adequately treated.

External bleeding

Haematuria and nose bleeds common — usually settle easily with treatment. Investigate for bleeding point if persistent. GI bleeding relatively unusual and often associated with underlying cause, e.g. piles, duodenal ulcer. Bleeding from tooth sockets will inevitably occur after extractions — often delayed and extremely persistent. Dental extractions should always be carried out under appropriate haemostatic cover.

Petechial haemorrhages are *not* a feature of haemophiliac bleeding.

Traumatic bleeding

Haemophiliacs bleed severely and persistently after trauma, though this may often be delayed for up to several hours or even days after the event. Surgery will similarly provoke bleeding even in mild haemophiliacs.

DIAGNOSTIC COAGULATION TESTS

1. Prolonged activated partial thromboplastin time (APTT, e.g. PTTK or KCCT).
2. Normal prothrombin time.
3. Normal bleeding time.
4. Normal platelets.
5. Reduced factor VIII or IX level on clotting assay (F VIII C, F IX C).
6. Prolonged whole blood clotting time (only in more severe cases and too inaccurate to be useful).
7. Additional tests for haemophilia A:
   a. Factor VIII related antigen (F VIII RAg). Immunological assay of the non-coagulant part of the factor VIII molecule. Normal in haemophiliacs
   b. Factor VIII pro-coagulant antigen (F VIII CAg). The immunological expression of the coagulant part of the factor VIII molecule. In 90% of haemophiliacs it parallels the F VIII C level. In the remaining 10% it is significantly higher.

NB: 1. It is essential in Haemophilia A to demonstrate the normal F VIII RAg in addition to the low F VIII C in order to distinguish it from von Willebrand's disease (see below).

2. Tests should be repeated preferably three times before the diagnosis is established and a level of severity documented. Partially clotted samples can for instance give falsely low coagulant values.

MANAGEMENT

In the United Kingdom all haemophiliacs should be registered with a Regional or Supraregional Haemophilia Centre and their management should be supervised from there. Haemophilia is a relatively uncommon disorder potentially causing great patient morbidity. Effective treatment is available but is expensive and appropriate management requires care and experience. Early treatment with appropriate blood products lessens morbidity and is relatively cost effective, and so a management system which allows the patient easy and quick access to treatment is extremely important. For these reasons the Regional Centres have been set up allowing direct self referral by the patient for bleeding episodes, and many patients are now on home treatment for the more straightforward bleeding problems. Regular review is important.

Many of the diagnostic assays are available only at specialized centres. Any hospital managing haemophiliacs should be able to carry out at least the coagulation assays. 'Associate centres' are linked to a regional centre and may manage the more day-to-day problems of haemophiliacs living in their area.

The following notes on management are for guidance only, and assume that the patient will be under the care of an appropriately trained haematologist. Many centres issue a handbook for junior staff which should be used if available.

Baseline investigations (see also 'complications' for rationale of these)

1. Diagnostic coagulation studies as above.
2. Inhibitor screen.
3. Full blood count — including platelets.
4. Liver function tests especially AST level.
5. Hepatitis B surface antigen and antibody.
6. Blood group and red cell antibody screen.
7. X-rays of chronically affected joints.
8. Others as indicated — e.g. any screening tests for non-A non-B hepatitis or AIDS that are, or may become, available.

Documentation

1. Easily accessible records with diagnosis, F VIII C and F VIII RAg levels should be kept, and a Haemophilia Card issued to the patient by the Haemophilia Centre.
2. All bleeding episodes and treatment given (including batch numbers) must be accurately recorded. Patients on home treatment must be instructed to keep their own records and hand them in when renewing supplies.
3. Family members should be recorded and seen for diagnosis and counselling where appropriate.

Therapeutic materials used

Blood products (see also Ch. 29)
1. Haemophilia A
   a. Cryoprecipitate: each pack contains from 30–100 units factor VIII in about 25 ml plasma
      Advantages:
      (i)   Single donor units hence low hepatitis and AIDS risk
      (ii) Relatively inexpensive
      Disadvantages:
      (i)   Individual packs not assayed, hence dose approximate only
      (ii) Relatively large volume
      (iii) Frozen at -20 to $-70°C$ so storage difficult especially for home treatment
      (iv) Allergic reactions more common than concentrate
   b. Factor VIII concentrate: produced in freeze dried form with exactly calculated dose on each bottle, to be made up with water
      Advantages:
      (i)   Able to give exact dose
      (ii) Convenient — small volume stored at 4°C or room temperature if necessary
      Disadvantages:
      (i)   A product pooled from many donations, hence relatively high hepatitis and AIDS risk.
2. Haemophilia B
   Factor IX concentrate (also contains factors II and X) is the only useful therapeutic material available.

Similar advantages and disadvantages to factor VIII concentrate. Also potentially thrombogenic therefore in most situations it is advisable to aim for less than total correction of the factor IX level, even for surgery.

Other therapeutic agents
1. Antifibrinolytic agents, e.g. tranexamic acid: prevents breakdown of clot once formed. Useful for surface bleeding e.g. nose bleeds, GI tract bleeding, tooth extractions.
   NB: Do not use for bleeding into confined spaces e.g. joints, urinary tract as damage from clot retention may occur.
   Dose: 25 mg/kg 8 hourly p.o. or 15 mg/kg 8 hourly i.v.
2. DDAVP (desamino d-arginine vasopressin).
   Vasopressin analogue which causes two to three fold rise in factor VIII level. Useful for relatively minor surgical procedures e.g. tooth extraction in patients with *mild* haemophilia A and von Willebrand's disease.

Given i.v. — usual dose 0.3 μg/kg prior to procedure. Should combine with i.v. and then oral tranexamic acid as DDAVP stimulates fibrinolysis.
Dose may be repeated 12 hourly for a few doses only as effect tends to be reduced after first injection. May cause headache and fluid retention.

Treatment

General

1. Do not use intramuscular injections at any time.
2. Drugs may be given orally, i.v. or subcutaneously.
3. Do not use aspirin as it will aggravate the bleeding tendency by interfering with platelet function.
4. Treat all bleeds as soon as possible with adequate amounts of factor VIII or IX.
5. Carefully preserve the patient's veins. Use non-traumatic 'butterfly' type needles whenever possible. Ensure haemostasis at venepuncture sites to prevent bruising.

Calculating the dose of factor VIII or IX

Different situations call for different levels of factor VIII or IX for adequate haemostasis and hence the dose given will depend on the type of bleed.

To calculate the appropriate dose the following formulae can be used:

$$\text{Factor VIII, number of units required} = \frac{\%\ \text{rise required x weight in kg}}{1.5}$$

$$\text{Factor IX, number of units required} = \frac{\%\ \text{rise required x weight in kg}}{0.7}$$

These will give approximate requirements only as some patients do not show a completely predictable rise.

The following is a *guide* to the levels to be aimed at in different bleeding situations in haemophilia A:

Type of bleeding	Levels of factor VIII desirable
Minor bleeding	10– 20%
Major bleeding or dental extraction	20– 50%
Surgery	50–100%

NB: In haemophilia B:

1. Levels may in general be allowed to fall a little below those of factor VIII in equivalent situation.
2. Do not aim to raise levels above 70–80% even for surgery as thrombosis may ensue.

Assays: for serious bleeding it is essential to check levels regularly before and after treatment to ensure that haemostatic levels are present at all times.

Frequency of treatment

Factor VIII: to maintain adequate levels at all times, e.g. for surgery, infusions will be required 8–12 hourly.

Factor IX: longer half life than factor VIII hence 12 hourly infusions adequate for maintaining levels.

For spontaneous bleeds, a single adequate infusion will often be sufficient, although more severe bleeds almost always require two treatments or more for resolution. Judgement about this depends on the patient's response to treatment and on experience.

Joint and soft tissue bleeds
1. Assessment
   a. Spontaneous or traumatic — if the latter more treatment likely to be needed
   b. Time elapsed since onset — if delayed more treatment likely to be needed
   c. Physical signs — swelling, warmth, immobility, signs of trauma
   d. In soft tissue bleeds check for signs of vascular or neurological compression
   e. Note severity of factor deficiency, and presence or absence of inhibitor.
2. Haemostasis
   Give 5–10 i.u./kg appropriate concentrate or cryoprecipitate by i.v. infusion.
3. General measures
   Rest, immobilization and relief from weight bearing. Bed rest may be necessary especially for lower limb bleeds. Back slabs may be useful. Do *not* immobilise any limb in a cylinder plaster as serious pressure effects may occur from continued bleeding and swelling.
4. Analgesia
   Requirements may range from nil to regular opiates e.g. pethidine by i.v. infusion. Adequate analgesia is essential and although opiate addiction can be a problem in occasional severe haemophiliacs it is unjustifiable to withhold these drugs in acute situations. Long term chronic pain should obviously be managed with non-addictive drugs
   Do not use aspirin derivatives.
5. Physiotherapy
   Very important after immobilisation, especially after knee bleeds. Essential to build up muscles with appropriate exercises to help to support the joint and attain maximum mobility. Liaise with physiotherapy department, and orthopaedic surgeon.
6. Further treatment
   If treated as an out-patient and bleed does not resolve on one infusion the patient should be asked to return for further doses. Serious lower limb bleeds or unresolving bleeds require admission for rest and regular treatment
   Any bleed in a site vulnerable from nerve or vascular damage, e.g. forearm, buttock or calf, or hand bleeds where joint damage can cause serious disability, require regular supervision until resolved.

Bleeds at other sites

1. GI tract — haematemesis or melaena.
   a. Admission mandatory
   b. Give 10–20 i.u./kg appropriate factor and monitor levels
   c. Give tranexamic acid (see above)
   d. Otherwise treat as any other patient with GIT haemorrhage (transfusion as necessary, endoscopy, cimetidine).
2. GU Tract
   a. If persistent give 5–10 units/kg appropriate factor
   b. Bed rest may be helpful
   c. *Do not* use antifibrinolytic drugs
   d. Culture urine, treat UTI
   e. Investigate for underlying lesion if persistent (X-ray abdomen, IVU).
3. CNS:
   a. Treat with great urgency
   b. Give sufficient factor VIII or IX as early as possible to achieve > 50% levels. Continue to keep levels haemostatic until bleed resolved
   c. CT scanning may be helpful in defining extent of bleed, and in picking up any underlying lesion
   d. Do not carry out lumbar puncture unless absolutely essential, and then only under full haemostatic cover.
4. Mouth, throat and neck
   Can cause serious complications, e.g. respiratory obstruction, if not treated adequately. Patient should be admitted and regular treatment given till resolved.

Dental care

1. Regular visits to dentist essential for careful conservation. Fillings may be carried out normally.
2. Local anaesthesia. Local gum infiltration may be used with care, but nerve blocks should not be given unless under haemostatic cover.
3. Extractions require haemostatic cover with assays. Check for inhibitor first. Levels of 20–50% necessary prior to operation. May be achieved with appropriate blood product, or in mild haemophilia with DDAVP. Avoid concentrate in haemophiliacs not previously exposed to it, if at all possible. Single dose often adequate, though for major work e.g. wisdom teeth, several infusions may be necessary.
4. Soft dental splints may reduce blood loss. Topical thrombin may be used for oozing but is no substitute for an adequate factor level.
5. Tranexamic acid and prophylactic antibiotics e.g. Penicillin V 250 mg q.d.s. should be given for approximately five days.

Surgery

1. Before any procedure check baseline factor level, screen for inhibitor and assess for carriage of hepatitis B. Blood group and antibody screen and cross match appropriate number of units.
   Liaise closely with all staff involved in the patient's care about the special needs of haemophiliacs.
2. Aim for levels of 50–100% in haemophilia A and 50–70% in haemophilia B. Use concentrate, cryoprecipitate or DDAVP as appropriate. The decision about which product to use is an expert one. Levels should always be checked pre and post infusion and an adequate level obtained before surgery commences.
3. Repeat infusions 8–12 hourly are required to keep levels haemostatic till healing has occurred. Such a regime should be planned by the haemophilia consultant.
4. Scrupulous operative technique and haemostasis are essential and the surgical management of haemophiliacs should wherever possible be left to a team which is closely involved with the haemophilia centre.

Complications

Long term joint damage
Very common, though should lessen as haemophiliacs receive better and earlier treatment for joint bleeds.

Affects particularly knees, ankles, elbows, shoulders, hips. Regular review in an orthopaedic clinic should be arranged.

Treatment:

1. Splinting and physiotherapy. Contact physiotherapy department. Physiotherapy to build up supporting muscle groups may lessen the frequency of bleeds.
2. Synovectomy — mainly for repeated knee bleeds, but occasionally other joints.
   Sometimes useful for repeated bleeds in a chronically swollen 'boggy' knee which retains good movement.
3. Joint replacement. Best results are in painful, stiff joints which are beyond the stage of frequent bleeding. Prosthetic joints are available for hips and in some centres knee and ankle replacements have been carried out. Results often excellent though further bleeding around the joint may be a problem. In young patients too there is the problem that the prosthetic joint is required to work well for many years, in contrast to the more routine total hip replacement in an elderly arthritic patient.
4. Arthrodesis. May be suitable for joints where there is a lot of pain on movement and already a loss of useful mobility. Often excellent for pain relief but the patient must accept that the joint will be completely rigid.

Liver disease

Most haemophiliacs on regular treatment with blood products develop abnormal biochemical tests of liver function, particularly elevation of transaminases (i.e. AST and ALT). Marked fluctuation in the levels may occur. Clinically there may be no abnormality at all, though episodes of acute hepatitis (usually non-A non-B in type, sometimes hepatitis B) are common, particularly in patients who have had no blood products previously and then receive factor concentrate. Histologically there is evidence of disease ranging from benign chronic persistent hepatitis to frank cirrhosis. Serological evidence of previous hepatitis B infection, or chronic carriage of hepatitis B antigen is common, and there is presumptive evidence that this is important in the development of deranged liver function, though other factors such as immune complex formation may be relevant.

Prevention:

1. Use DDAVP or cryoprecipitate for mild haemophiliacs in preference to concentrate. Try to limit the number of batches of concentrate to which any patient is exposed, as this reduces the potential exposure to infectious agents.
2. Steriods may be indicated if histology suggests chronic active hepatitis — liver biopsy is justifiable if there is a possibility that treatment may be based on the result.

Acquired immune deficiency syndrome

AIDS has been seen in a number of haemophiliacs, mainly so far in the United States of America. The disease presents with persistent lymphadenopathy, and opportunistic infections, and in haemophiliacs is probably related to HTLV III (p. 122) infection acquired from blood products. Limiting exposure to concentrates where possible presumably reduces the risk. Newly available heat treated concentrates should be virus-free.

Inhibitor formation

Approximately 10% of patients with severe haemophilia A develop inhibitors to factor VIII after treatment. These inhibitors are antibodies to factor VIII CAg. They may appear after relatively little treatment, and once present will tend to be boosted by further treatment with factor VIII. They may be suspected clinically by failure of the patient to respond to treatment or in vitro by lack of rise in factor VIII levels after treatment, or failure of the patient's prolonged APTT to correct with normal plasma. The inhibitor titre may be quantified in vitro.

Clinically they make treatment much more difficult, especially if present in high titre. They do not however increase the frequency of bleeds.

Management of inhibitor patients

This is difficult and expensive and requires expert supervision.

1. Regular checks on severe haemophiliacs for the presence of an inhibitor — essential prior to elective procedures.

2. Larger than usual doses of factor VIII may neutralise the inhibitor and allow haemostasis. Often the clinical effect is better than would be predicted from the rise in the factor VIII level. Doses required may be many times normal. Boosting of the inhibitor from treatment usually begins from about five days after treatment and levels should be regularly checked. It is important when using human factor VIII to overcome an inhibitor that resolution of the bleed is achieved within these few days.
3. Factor IX concentrates or activated products such as 'FEIBA' may be used to bypass factor VIII in the coagulation pathway and hence achieve haemostasis. Dosage and monitoring very difficult and products very expensive.
4. Porcine factor VIII. Recent concentrates produced by new techniques give good haemostasis without the problem of thrombocytopenia seen with previous animal products. Very effective for relatively low titre antibodies but expensive and patients may develop porcine antibodies thus rendering them progressively less effective. Severe anaphylactic reactions occasionally occur.

Genetics

Sex linked disorders, therefore:
1. Daughters of haemophiliacs are obligatory carriers.
2. Sons of haemophiliacs are normal.
3. Sons of carriers have 50/50 chance of being affected.
4. Daughters of carriers have 50/50 chance of being carriers.

Many known carriers do not wish to risk producing a severely affected haemophiliac child, and antenatal diagnosis may be offered as follows to known or probable carriers:
1. Amniocentesis at 16–18 weeks to sex the child.
2. Fetal blood sampling if fetus male, to measure F VIII C, CAg and RAg, or in haemophilia B the FIX level.
3. Current research suggests that analysis of chorionic DNA may prove to be the diagnostic method of choice.

Detection of carriers

Most carriers have some reduction in the F VIII C and CAg level relative to the F VIII RAg level though great variability exists. C/RAg ratios should be measured on at least three occasions and the results computed together with the genetic probability in order to produce a final probability of being a carrier. The diagnosis cannot be predicted with full certainty. DNA analysis may be the future method of choice.

VON WILLEBRAND'S DISEASE

Autosomally dominant inherited bleeding disorder arising from complex and variable abnormalities of the non-coagulant part of the factor VIII molecule. This larger part of the factor VIII complex includes factor VIII RAg activity and also interacts with platelets during normal haemostasis. The functional effect on platelet interaction can be demonstrated in vitro by its action as a co-factor (F VIII RiCOF) during platelet aggregation with ristocetin.

As the F VIII RiCOF or von Willebrand factor complexes in vivo with F VIII C, low levels of F VIII C may be demonstrated in most patients even though they are able to synthesize it normally.

This biochemically complex disease is associated with any combination of the following abnormalities:

1. Prolonged bleeding time.
2. Reduced F VIII C.
3. Reduced F VIII RAg.
4. Abnormalities of F VIII RAg in its quantity or molecular size distribution demonstrated by electrophoresis.
5. Reduced F VIII RiCOF as demonstrated by platelet aggregation with ristocetin.

Clinical features

Very variable but seldom a very severe bleeding disorder in comparison to haemophilia, except in occasional homozygote patients. Affects sexes equally. Mild cases may escape detection till well into adulthood. Patients should be registered with a haemophilia centre.

Type of bleeding

1. Bleeding tends to be more superficial in nature than in haemophilia with joint bleeds much less common.
2. Nose bleeds, gum bleeding, menorrhagia and easy bruising common.
3. Bleeding on trauma, or after dental extraction or surgery.

Treatment

1. A single infusion of factor VIII in any form will produce an initial rise and then a second prolonged peak in VIII C levels. Treatment thus produces haemostatic levels for 24–48 hours and hence frequent treatment unnecessary in most cases, even for surgery. Cryoprecipitate is the best form in which to give the factor VIII.
2. Many bleeding episodes are mild and may not need any other than local treatment, e.g. contraceptive pill for menorrhagia.
3. DDAVP and/or an antifibrinolytic drug are useful as in haemophilia.

4. The usual method of monitoring treatment is by means of F VIII C assays, as although it would be more logical to measure F VIII RiCOF, the F VIII C assay is much simpler.
5. Calculating the dose of factor VIII is rather more empirical than in haemophilia but in general good haemostasis is easily achieved.
6. Management of surgery and dental work is similar to that of haemophiliacs.

REFERENCES

Biggs R 1974 Recent advances in the management of haemophilia and Christmas disease. Clinics in Haematolgoy 8(1): 95–105
Bloom A L, Peake I R 1977 F VIII and its related disorders. British Medical Bulletin 33(3): 219–224
Rizza C R 1977 Clinical management of haemophilia. British Medical Bulletin 33: 225–230
Zimmerman T S, Ruggeri Z M 1983 von Willebrand's disease. Clinics in Haematology 12(1): 83–95

Part 7
TRANSFUSION

29. BLOOD COMPONENT THERAPY

Single donor units of blood are commonly split into separate components to allow more appropriate and efficient treatment of specific deficiencies.

RED CELLS

In general red cell transfusion should be avoided if alternative methods of treatment for anaemia are appropriate (e.g. iron or B12 therapy). Although compatibility testing matches donor and recipient for ABO and Rhesus D antigens, it is impossible to match for all the minor red cell antigens (e.g. c̄, Kell, Duffy) and sensitisation may occur with the production of antibodies that make subsequent transfusion difficult. Because of the risk of haemolytic disease of the newborn (p.   ) it is important not to risk sensitising women of child-bearing age. Also hepatitis (B and non-A/non-B) and AIDS transmission may occur.

Stored whole blood

Constituents
1. Red cells.
2. Plasma proteins, particularly albumin.
3. Small amount of fibrinogen.

NB: Contains no therapeutic amounts of other clotting factors, and no viable platelets or granulocytes.

Indication
1. Acute blood loss, particularly volume replacement of more than one litre.

Storage
1. 4°C in hospital blood bank. Must not be removed from refrigerator more than 30 minutes before transfusion.
2. Depending on anticoagulant used, red cells remain viable for up to five weeks.

Plasma reduced/packed cells/concentrated red cells

Constituents

      1. Red cells. Plasma has been removed from the pack, either at the Blood Transfusion Centre or in the hospital blood bank, to give an haematocrit of 60–65% for plasma reduced blood, or a selected higher haematocrit for packed cells/concentrated cells.

Indications

      1. Bone marrow failure e.g. aplastic anaemia, leukaemia. In the treatment of anaemia one unit of packed cells should raise the haemoglobin by approximately 1g/dl in adults.

      2. Chronic persistent blood loss, especially when Hb < 7g/dl.

      3. Haemolysis

          a. Congenital haemoglobinopathies e.g. ß-thalassaemia major — usually require regular transfusion (p. 36), sickle cell anaemia — less need for regular transfusion (Ch. 7). May need leucocyte depleted blood if non-haemolytic transfusion reactions are troublesome (see below)

          b. Immune-mediated haemolysis. In warm auto-immune haemolytic anaemia cross-matching may be difficult because of the patients positive direct antiglobulin (Coombs) test; even the patients own red cells appear incompatible with his serum. It is usually necessary to select the least incompatible from a selection of units to transfuse. In cold auto-immune haemolytic anaemia use an in-line blood warmer if possible.

Storage

As for whole blood (above) but if plasma has been removed in hospital blood bank use within 12 hours.

Leucocyte-depleted blood

Leucocytes may be removed by centrifuging the blood pack to compact the buffy coat layer and then using an in-line microaggregate filter at the patients bedside. More efficient removal may be achieved by special filtration, saline washing, or using frozen and reconstituted red cells (all these procedures are done at the blood transfusion centre).

Constituents

      1. Red cells.

      2. Suspending medium — usually saline.

Indication

      1. Prevention or amelioration of non-haemolytic transfusion reactions demonstrated to be due to leucocyte antibodies in the recipient.

Storage

      1. After preparation stored at 4°C until use.

      2. Usually must be used within 12 hours of preparation, expiry time indicated on pack.

Frozen red cells

Constituents
1. Red cells uncontaminated by other cells or plasma.
2. Suspending solution, commonly saline.

Indications
1. Supply of very rare blood groups. Individuals with these groups may have their red cells frozen for future use.
2. Preparation of fully leucocyte-depleted red cells. Used when other, less efficient, methods of leucocyte removal have still resulted in febrile reactions.

Storage
1. Last indefinitely in frozen state.
2. When thawed and washed of cryopreservative must be used within 12 hours.

Fresh blood

Blood used within 24 hours of donation. Because expedited testing and processing techniques required, the use of fresh blood is usually restricted to the transfusion of neonates. There is a higher risk of transmitting cytomegalovirus (CMV) infection with fresh blood than stored blood.

Constituents
1. Red cells.
2. Viable platelets.
3. Small amounts of all coagulation factors.
4. Plasma proteins (if not plasma reduced).

Indications
1. Top-up and exchange transfusion of neonates, often used as 'baby fresh O Negative' for the treatment of Rhesus haemolytic disease (p. 35).
2. Occasionally has been used in the rare patient who requires all the constituents of fresh blood. This can be now more efficiently achieved using specific component therapy.

PLATELETS

Platelet concentrates (in 30–40 ml plasma) are prepared from single units of blood. These may be issued as single packs or pooled for convenience.

Sources
1. Random donor.
2. Plateletpheresis pack obtained from a single donor using a cell separator, issued as platelet rich plasma. Equivalent to six single units of platelet concentrate.

3. Single, HLA matched. Obtained as in 2., but either from selected HLA matched unrelated donor or family member. The latter should be avoided if bone marrow transplantation is contemplated.

Indications

1. Prophylactic. Usually used with transient and predictable bone marrow suppression e.g. after cytotoxic drug therapy. Not recommended as a routine for chronic thrombocytopenia not associated with bleeding, because of the danger of alloimmunisation resulting in destruction of transfused platelets without clinical benefit. Generally infusions are given daily, or on alternate days. Aim to keep platelet count $> 20 \times 10^9/1$, by giving one unit of platelet concentrate per 10kg body weight.
2. For bleeding associated with thrombocytopenia:
   a. Bone marrow suppression or infiltration
   b. Dilution with massive transfusion
   c. Extra corporeal circulation e.g. coronary bypass
   d. Inherited and acquired disorders of platelet function.

Platelet transfusion is usually ineffective in disorders associated with immune destruction of platelets e.g. ITP (p.   ), post transfusion purpura. In these disorders platelet transfusion is usually only used to cover operations (e.g. splenectomy in ITP) or acute life-threatening bleeding. When resistance to transfused platelets is due to alloimmunisation use HLA matched platelets (see above).

Constituents

1. Platelets.
2. Small amounts of all coagulation factors and plasma proteins — the platelets are suspended in fresh plama.
3. Contaminating leucocytes — may cause non-haemolytic febrile transfusion reactions.
4. Contaminating red cells — give ABO and Rhesus compatible platelets when possible. If it is necessary to give Rhesus positive donor platelets to a Rhesus negative recipient consider giving anti-D 500 i.u. i.m./s.c. to prevent Rhesus (D) immunisation.

Storage

1. Function preserved best when stored at room temperature.
2. Continuous gentle agitation during storage helps prevent clumping.
3. Usually must be used within 72 hours of preparation — observe expiry time on pack.

WHITE CELLS

Sources

1. Random donor buffy coat preparations. Usually require at least 12 units to achieve a therapeutically effective dose.
2. Single donor leucapheresis pack. Obtained (using cell separator from healthy donor, or patient with CGL (p.   ).
3. HLA matched leucapheresis donor. Used when reaction to granulocytes is thought to be due to HLA antibodies.

Constituents

1. Granulocytes. A minimum therapeutic dose is generally estimated to be 5×10^{11} granulocytes (or 5×10^{10} if HLA matched).
2. Lymphocytes. It is usual to irradiate the pack before infusion into the recipient to prevent possible graft-versus-host disease.
3. Platelets — may be therapeutic if patient is also thrombocytopenic.
4. Red cells — use ABO and Rhesus compatible donors, and cross-match donor red cells with recipients serum.
5. Small amounts of fresh plasma.

Indications

1. Proven infections in granulocytopenic ($< 0.5 \times 10^9/1$ neutrophils) patients whose fever is unresponsive to 48 hours treatment with appropriate broad spectrum antibiotics. Generally the granulocytopenia is of a temporary nature, e.g. post cytotoxic marrow hypoplasia, drug idiosyncrasy. The efficacy of granulocyte transfusions is unproven.

Storage

Use immediately.

PLASMA PROTEINS

Plasma protein fraction (PPF)

Constituents

1. Albumin in 4.5 g/dl concentration (iso-osmotic with plasma).
2. Electrolytes (Na 150mmol/l, K < 2.0 mmol/1).

NB: No clotting factors or gamma globulin.

Indications

1. Volume replacement in acute haemorrhage whilst awaiting compatible blood.
2. Burns — lose massive amounts of protein in exudate.
3. As a replacement fluid in plasma exchange.

Storage
1. Room temperature in dark.
2. Shelf life of two years, as has been pasteurised during manufacture — no risk of hepatitis transmission.

Salt-poor albumin

Constituents
1. Albumin in 20g/dl concentration (hypertonic with respect to plasma).
2. Very small amounts of sodium relative to protein concentration (Na < 140mmol/l, K < 2mmol/l).

Indications
1. Severe hypoproteinaemia with oedema due to nephrotic syndrome, in order to increase circulating blood volume (by osmotically attracting fluid into the circulation from the extracellular space) and establish a diuresis.
2. Severe hypoproteinaemia with oedema due to liver failure. Probably a waste of time to administer chronically, but may be useful to cover acute clinical events.

Administration of salt poor albumin in these situations is of temporary benefit only. 1 × 100ml bottle will raise the serum albumin in an adult by approximately 5g/1.

Storage
As for PPF (see above)

Fresh frozen plasma (FFP)

Constituents
1. Normal amounts of all clotting factors.
2. Plasma proteins.
3. Blood group antibodies and contaminating red cell fragments. Give ABO and Rhesus compatible units or group AB Rhesus negative FFP.
4. Citrate anticoagulant.

Indications
1. A source of clotting factors for the treatment of DIC (p. 175) and haemodilution with stored blood (p. 177). In the latter it is usual to give one unit of FFP for every 5–6 units of rapidly transfused banked blood.
2. The treatment of clotting factor deficiencies when the exact factor deficiency has not been established, or when more appropriate clotting factor concentrates are not immediately available.

3. As source of pseudocholinesterase in patients who fail to recover spontaneously from suxamethonium induced paralysis due to a congenital deficiency of pseudocholinesterase.
4. As a supplement or alternative to PPF in plasma exchange therapy.

Storage

1. Stored frozen. At −40°C usual shelf life is six months.
2. After thawing (by placing in a water bath at 37°C), should be used immediately.

Cryoprecipitate

Constituents

1. Factor VIII and fibrinogen and fibronectin.
2. ABO antibodies and contaminating red cell fragments. Give ABO and (ideally) Rhesus compatible units.

Indications

1. Treatment of haemophilia A (p. 193).
2. Treatment of DIC (p.   ), and fibrinogen deficiency.

Storage

As for FFP (see above).

Coagulation factor concentrates

Constituents

1. Both factor VIII and factor IX concentrates are available.

Indications

1. Treatment of haemophilia A and Christmas disease (Ch. 28).

Storage

1. At 4°C in dark
2. Use immediately once reconstituted.

REFERENCES

Hollan S A 1981 Controversial and changing trends in blood transfusion. Vox Sanguinis 40: 309–316
Urbaniak S J, Cash J D 1977 Blood replacement therapy. British Medical Bulletin 33(3): 273–282

30. ACUTE TRANSFUSION REACTIONS

DEFINITION

Any untoward response to blood or blood products occurring during, or shortly after transfusion.

Other complications of transfusion, of a more delayed nature, are dealt with in Ch. 29.

HAEMOLYTIC REACTION

This results from antibodies directed against red cell antigens causing haemolysis in the recipient. Generally the most immediate, serious and severe type of transfusion reaction. If, however, the haemolysis is mainly extra-vascular, due to a non-complement-fixing antibody, then the only signs may be post transfusion jaundice and anaemia (Fig. 30.1).

Causes

1. ABO mismatched transfusion, usually due to clerical error, or failure to correctly identify patient. May be fatal.
2. Antibodies in recipients plasma against minor red cell antigens on donor red cells. Usually preventable by adequate cross-matching of donor cells with recipients plasma.
3. Administration of blood that has been haemolysed before transfusion due to inadvertent freezing, heating, infection or use of grossly out-dated blood.
4. Antibodies in the donors plasma reacting with the recipients red cells. Relatively mild reactions most common with administration of 'high-titre' group 0 whole blood or plasma to group A or B recipients. Avoided by screening out group 0 donors with strong anti-A or Anti-B, and using packed cells rather than whole blood.

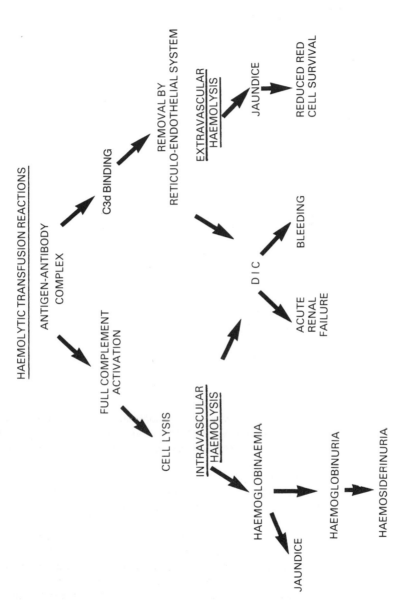

Fig. 30.1 Mechanism of haemolytic transfusion reaction

Clinical features

Reaction usually occurs within 30 minutes of starting transfusion, sometimes when only a small amount of blood has been transfused.

1. Pain at drip site, in loins and chest.
2. Pyrexia and rigors.
3. Hypotension, tachycardia, shock. Usually peripheral vasoconstriction, but vasodilatation if due to infected blood.
4. Haemoglobinuria.
5. Bleeding manifestations of DIC. With hypotension may be the only indication of a haemolytic reaction in patients under general anaesthesia.

Laboratory investigations

1. Inspection of plasma and urine for free haemoglobin, naked-eye and by spectroscope. Schumm's test for methaemalbumin (free haemoglobin binds to albumin) in plasma.
2. Re-group and re-cross-match patient and the donor units using a fresh blood sample taken from the opposite arm to the drip site.
3. Culture and gram-stain donor units for bacteria. Blood-culture from recipient.
4. Direct antiglobulin (Coomb's) test on patient's blood.
5. Haemoglobin, coagulation screen and platelet count to look for DIC.
6. Electrolyte and urea measurement.

Management

1. *Stop the transfusion immediately*. Send samples for tests indicated above to the laboratory.
2. Maintain blood pressure and circulating blood volume by infusion of PPF (p. 209) or crystalloid solutions, preferably monitoring by measurement of central venous pressure (CVP) to avoid circulatory overload.
3. Monitor urine output closely, and attempt to prevent tubular necrosis by administration of diuretic, e.g. 100ml of 20% mannitol (plus optimum hydration with saline), frusemide 40–120mg i.v.
4. Correct electrolyte abnormalities, e.g. hyperkalaemia, as appropriate.
5. Treat the coagulation abnormalities of DIC with FFP and platelet concentrate as appropriate.
6. If infected blood is suspected administer broad spectrum antibiotic.

7. If acute renal failure supervenes (indicated by urine output < 30ml/hr, urinary urea < 160mmol/l, urinary sodium > 20mmol/l — i.e. approaching those of plasma) restrict fluid and consult renal physician with a view to early dialysis.

NON-HAEMOLYTIC FEBRILE REACTION

The commonest type of immediate transfusion reaction.

Causes

1. Leucocyte or platelet antibodies in recipient due to previous immunisation by transfusion or pregnancy.
2. Sensitivity to foreign proteins in transfused blood.
3. Unidentified pyrogens in transfused fluids or giving set.

Clinical features

1. Pyrexia, shivering, rigors. Commonly 30 minutes — 3 hours after start of transfusion.
2. Malaise, headache.

Management

1. Stop the transfusion. Maintain infusion with saline.
2. If reaction does not settle promptly, or if clinical features of haemolysis (above) are present then investigate as for haemolytic reaction.
3. Aspirin may provide symptomatic relief if not contra-indicated because of impairment of platelet function. Administration of hydrocortisone is usually unnecessary.
4. If reaction settles continue cautiously with next unit of blood.
5. Arrange for leucocyte antibody investigations.
6. Consult the laboratory about obtaining leucocyte poor blood (p. 206) should further transfusions be necessary.

ALLERGIC REACTION

Causes

1. Anti-IgA antibodies in recipients with congenital deficiency of IgA. Usually anaphylactic type reaction.
2. Antibodies against variable antigenic determinants on IgG (Gm) and IgA.
3. Commonly there is an atopic history (asthma, hayfever, eczema).

Clinical features

Clinical features of febrile reaction (see above) may also be present.

1. Skin rashes, urticaria.
2. Wheezing and bronchospasm.
3. Angioneurotic oedema.
4. Anaphylaxis (a severe reaction involving the above features with circulatory collapse).

Management

1. Stop transfusion. Maintain infusion with saline.
2. Administer antihistamine, e.g. chlorpheniramine 10mg slow i.v.
3. If severe then give hydrocortisone 100–200mg i.v. The more severe reactions require investigation before further transfusion — discuss with the haematologist.
4. When settled continue transfusion cautiously with next unit. Adrenaline 1ml of 1 in 1000 s.c. may be necessary for anaphylaxis.

CIRCULATORY OVERLOAD

Causes

1. Existing heart disease.
2. Elderly patients.
3. Chronic anaemia, particularly megaloblastic.
4. Overenthusiastic infusion rate.

Clinical features

1. Basal crepitations, upper lobe diversion and raised jugular venous pressure.
2. Acute left ventricular failure with dyspnoea, cyanosis, frothy sputum.

Management

1. Prevent by using packed cells, diuretic cover, e.g. frusemide 20–40mg i.v., transfuse slowly, monitor CVP if line available. As a general rule 1 unit of plasma reduced red cells may be transfused over two hours in the young adult; four to six hours in the elderly.
2. If congestive heart failure develops then stop transfusion, give diuretics, venesect if necessary.

AIR EMBOLISM

The introduction of air into the circulation. Small bubbles of air within the drip tubing (< 2ml) are clinically insignificant.

Causes

1. Raising the air pressure within a bottle of transfusion fluid to speed infusion, then allowing the drip to run through.
2. Disconnection of a central venous pressure line at the hub, or splitting between cannula and hub.
3. Inexpert use of extra-corporeal circulation with pump assistance, e.g. cell separator.
4. Other causes, e.g. failure to run fluid through giving set prior to infusion.

Clinical features

1. Chest pain and constriction, cough, shortness of breath. Mill-wheel cardiac murmur.
2. Cyanosis.
3. If severe, hypotension, tachycardia and circulatory collapse.

Management

1. Lie patient on left side, head down, for two hours to allow air to gather in right ventricular apex, and be absorbed.
2. Administer oxygen as necessary.

MASSIVE TRANSFUSION OF STORED BLOOD

Stored banked blood administered rapidly in volumes greater than six units may cause:
1. Bleeding due to lack of platelets and coagulation factors in stored blood (see p.   for management).
2. Hypothermia, as blood is stored at 4°C: use a blood warmer.
3. Pulmonary microembolisation due to aggregates of fibrin with dead leucocytes and platelets in banked blood (shock lung). Use a micro-aggregate filter.
4. Hyperkalaemia. Unlikely if renal function is normal and infusion rate < 100ml/min.
5. Hypocalcaemic tetany (rare) due to citrate anticoagulant chelating recipient's plasma calcium. Give calcium gluconate (10mls 10%) slowly i.v.

REFERENCE

Mollison P L 1983 Blood transfusion in clinical medicine, 7th edn. Blackwell, Oxford, p 729–780

Part 8
SPECIAL CLINICAL SITUATIONS

31. PERINATAL HAEMATOLOGY

NORMAL BABY

Note that neonates have a different (and rapidly changing) set of normal haematological values compared to adults.

Haemoglobin

Normal neonates have a haemoglobin of 14–20 g/dl (depending on timing of cord clamping). The haemoglobin rises in the first day of life, then drops to its lowest level at nine weeks (10–11 g/dl). Macrocytosis present at birth gradually resolves; by nine weeks the MCV is in the adult range. At birth three-quarters of haemoglobin is HbF. The percentage of HbF drops at a rate of 3% per week to a level of 3% at six months when the majority of haemoglobin is HbA.

Blood film

Polychromasia, a high reticulocyte count, anisopoikilocytosis, target cells and nucleated red cells are seen in the normal neonate. By the sixth day nucleated red cells disappear from the blood and the reticulocyte count returns to normal.

White cells

Leucocytosis with left shift is normal. Neutrophils predominate at birth, then lymphocytes are the major population from two weeks to four years.

Red cell enzymes

Many red cell enzymes have low levels at birth. An important exception is G6PD which is higher in neonates.

IMPORTANT CAUSES OF ANAEMIA IN THE NEONATE

Haemorrhage

This may be visible — from the cord or gastrointestinal tract, or internal — retroperitoneal or cerebral. Feto-maternal haemorrhage may be detected by the Kleihauer (fetal-cell) test on maternal blood. Repeated venepuncture contributes to anaemia in infants with a small blood volume.

Prematurity

Premature infants have lower haemoglobins, higher reticulocyte counts and more nucleated red cells in the blood than full-term infants, and the degree of anaemia is proportional to gestation.

Decreased red cell survival

1. Congenital and acquired infections may cause decreased red cell survival as well as bone marrow depression.
2. Isoimmune haemolytic disease of the newborn (Ch. 6) may be detected by the direct Coomb's (antiglobulin) test on the baby's red cells and red cell antibody screen on maternal serum.
3. Enzyme defects, most common of which is G6PD deficiency especially in the presence of certain oxidising drugs (p. 38).
4. Alpha chain disorders, e.g. alpha thalassaemia trait (Ch. 2) (but not beta chain disorders such as beta thalassaemia, sickle cell disease).

Marrow hypoplasia

e.g. Diamond-Blackfan anaemia (pure red cell aplasia).

BLEEDING DISORDERS IN THE NEONATE

Investigation

Prothrombin time (PT), activated partial thromboplastin time (APPT), thrombin time (TT), fibrinogen level, platelet count. FDPs if DIC is suspected.

Important causes

1. Haemorrhagic disease of the newborn:
   Usually affects breast fed infants 2–3 days after delivery, particularly if premature. It is exacerbated by maternal antibiotic therapy prior to delivery and maternal consumption of anticonvulsants and coumarin anticoagulants.
   Investigations show prolonged PT, prolonged APPT, and frequently a prolonged TT. Platelet count and fibrinogen normal. Treatment is vitamin K (phytomenadione) 1mg i.m. or i.v. which is given prophylactically in many units.

2. Liver disease:
   Including hepatitis, hereditary fructose intolerance, galactosaemia.
   Suspect if infant has hepatomegaly, prolonged jaundice and abnormalities of liver function tests.
   Investigations show a similar picture to haemorrhagic disease of the newborn associated with decreased fibrinogen and moderate thrombocytopenia.

3. Thrombocytopenia:
   Many causes, e.g. maternal anti-platelet antibodies crossing the placenta; suspect particularly when there is a maternal history of ITP (treated or untreated) or SLE. Congenital infections such as toxoplasma, rubella and cytomegalovirus may also cause thrombocytopenia.
   A low platelet count is usually the only abnormality in the clotting screen.
   Treatment, if required, may include platelet concentrate and steroids, exchange transfusion and high dose intravenous gamma globulin.

4. Congenital clotting factor deficiencies:
   Check for family history of these disorders. Results of investigations will depend on which factor is missing (Ch. 28).

5. DIC:
   Usually the baby will have been obviously ill before the onset of haemorrhagic symptoms, particularly with sepsis and hypoxia.
   Thrombocytopenia is invariably present, and usually all coagulation test results are abnormal, with high levels of FDPs.
   Management involves treatment of the underlying cause and giving FFP and platelet concentrate as appropriate (p. 207).

REFERENCE

Glader B E (ed) 1978 Perinatal haematology. Clinics in Haematology 7(1)

32. HAEMATOLOGY OF PREGNANCY

NORMAL PREGNANCY

The following haematological changes occur in normal pregnancy:
1. Blood volume
   Increase in red cell mass of 20–30%
   Increase in plasma volume of 50%
   The net dilutional effect, maximal at 32 weeks, leads to an apparent anaemia. A haemoglobin below 10g/dl at any stage of pregnancy is probably abnormal.
2. Bone marrow
   Extremely active marrow which is easily suppressed by relatively mild chronic disease, e.g. urinary infection.
3. Haematinic assays
   Serum iron, B12, folate and ferritin all fall gradually during pregnancy, and TIBC rises. Diagnosis of nutritional anaemia is therefore more difficult particularly as blood film changes are often not marked. Red cell folate is a more reliable guide to deficiency than serum folate.
4. Coagulation system
   Normal pregnancy results in increased levels of fibrinogen, and other coagulation factors, often with raised FDPs. Fibrinolysis is impaired.

CAUSES OF ANAEMIA IN PREGNANCY

Physiological (see above).
Iron deficiency (p. 9).
Folate deficiency (p. 17).
Infection — especially chronic urinary tract infection.
Exaggeration of pre-existing anaemia by physiological dilution e.g. thalassaemia trait, sickle cell disease.
Other medical conditions e.g. renal failure, bleeding.
Primary haematological problems e.g. leukaemia, aplastic anaemia.

TREATMENT OF ANAEMIA IN PREGNANCY

Because of the iron requirements of the baby all pregnant women should take iron supplements (e.g. ferrous sulphate 200 mg daily)). Many clinics also provide folic acid in a combined tablet with iron (e.g. 'Co-Ferol' — ferrous fumarate 120mg + folic acid 200μg — 1 tablet daily). For the treatment of iron or folate deficiency these doses are insufficient and should be doubled or trebled. The treatment of iron deficiency and other anaemias is covered in appropriate chapters.

BLEEDING DISORDERS IN PREGNANCY

The management of DIC which may be caused by obstetric conditions such as abruptio placentae, amniotic fluid embolus, retained dead fetus, severe pre-eclampsia, or septic abortion is dealt with in Chapter 25.

Immune thrombocytopenic purpura (which frequently affects women of child-bearing age) may present during pregnancy and is considered in Chapter 11.

THROMBO-EMBOLIC PROBLEMS IN PREGNANCY

Increased coagulation factor levels and stasis in leg veins due to pressure of the enlarged uterus on inferior vena cava and iliac veins leads to increased incidence of thromboembolic problems, dealt with in Chapter 26. Elevated levels of FDPs are seen in pre-eclamptic toxaemia.

REFERENCE

Letsky E 1976 Haematological disease and pregnancy. British Journal of Hospital Medicine 15: 357–372

33. HAEMATOLOGICAL EFFECTS OF LIVER DISEASE

RED CELL MORPHOLOGY

Usually secondary to changes in plasma lipids affecting lipid structure in the red cell membrane.
1. Macrocytes
   a. Round' in liver disease or direct toxic effect of alcohol
   b. 'Oval' in folate or B12 deficiency.
2. Target cells (particularly in obstructive jaundice).
3. Stomatocytes.
4. Spur cells.
5. Dimorphic red cells (folate/B12 plus iron deficiency; alcohol induced sideroblastic anaemia).

CAUSES OF ANAEMIA

It is usually mild and multifactorial.
1. Iron deficiency: alcoholic diet, bleeding from low platelets, coagulopathy, portal hypertension, alcoholic gastritis.
2. Folate deficiency: particularly with alcohol excess (poor diet, anti-folate effect, vomiting).
3. B12 deficiency: unusual. May be seen in chronic alcoholic liver disease (prolonged poor diet, gastritis, damage to ileal mucosa). Damaged liver cells release stored B12 leading to high serum levels.
4. Hypoproliferative marrow: viral hepatitis, alcohol.
5. Haemolysis
   a. Portal hypertension causing hypersplenism (p. 91)
   b. Abnormal red cell membrane, e.g. spur cells
   c. Zieve's syndrome — acute fatty liver and hypertriglyceridaemia.
6. Dilutional: increased plasma volume in hypersplenism.

OTHER HAEMATOLOGICAL FEATURES OF LIVER DISEASE

1. Thrombocytopenia and leucopenia: toxic effect of alcohol, hypersplenism, viral hepatitis, folate deficiency.
2. Leucocytosis: viral hepatitis, metastatic carcinoma (Ch. 5).
3. Thrombocytosis: secondary carcinoma in liver, bleeding.
4. Polycythaemia: hepatoma.
5. Primary haematological disease resulting in hepatic dysfunction: thalassaemia major, sickle cell disease, Gaucher's disease, some leukaemias, lymphoma. Hyperbilirubinaemia due to haemolysis.

COAGULOPATHY IN LIVER DISEASE (See Ch. 25)

Causes
1. Thrombocytopenia. Lipid-induced abnormal platelet function.
2. Liver cell failure:
   a. Reduced synthesis of Vitamin K-dependent factors
   b. Reduced synthesis of factors V, VIII, anti-thrombin III and fibrinogen
   c. DIC — acute (acute hepatic necrosis) or chronic (impaired clearance of activated clotting factors)
   d. Dysfibrinogenaemia
   e. Increased fibrinolysis.

Investigation
1. Platelet count.
2. Prothrombin time: variably prolonged in any significant liver dysfunction. Good correlation with clinical outcome in paracetamol poisoning and hepatic pre-coma.
3. Thrombin time: sensitive to DIC and dysfibrinogenaemia.
4. APPT: variably prolonged.

Management
The likelihood of bleeding correlates poorly with the results of coagulation tests. The most common sites of bleeding are the gastrointestinal tract and venepuncture sites. Correction of the clotting times by administration of Vitamin K (most helpful in obstructive liver disease) and fresh frozen plasma is usually only partial. Liver biopsy in such patients is fraught with hazards.

REFERENCES

Roberts N R, Cederbaum A L 1972 The liver and blood coagulation physiology and pathology. Gastroentrology 63: 297–320
Zieve L 1966 Haemolytic anaemia in liver disease. Medicine 45: 497–505

34. HAEMATOLOGICAL EFFECTS OF RENAL DISEASE

The haematological abnormalities vary widely according to the nature of the renal disorder and the severity and chronicity of renal failure when present.

ANAEMIA OF RENAL FAILURE

Normochromic, normocytic anaemia often marked (Hb 5–9 g/dl) in established renal failure. The anaemia is usually most pronounced in anephric patients on haemodialysis; patients on continuous ambulatory peritoneal dialysis usually maintain a higher Hb than patients on haemodialysis.

Causes

1. Reduced production of red cells:
   a. Reduced erythropoietin production secondary to reduced functioning renal mass
   b. Toxic suppression of bone marrow by retention compounds.
2. Increased destruction of red cells:
   a. Impaired red cell metabolism and membrane function due to accumulation of toxic compounds
   b. Microangiopathy seen in some disorders
   c. Splenic destruction of those abnormal red cells causes hypersplenism which leads to further red cell destruction
   d. Mechanical damage from haemodialysis. Rarely, abnormal constituents or temperature of the dialysate.
3. Iron deficiency:
   a. Frequent venepuncture
   b. Blood loss in haemodialyser tubing
   c. Nutritional deficiency (low protein diet and poor appetite)
   d. Haematuria.
4. Folate deficiency:
   a. Poor nutrition
   b. Loss in dialysis fluid.

5. Dilutional:
   a. Increased plasma volume due to fluid retention and hypersplenism.

Treatment

1. Folic acid replacement (5 mg twice-weekly is sufficient) to patients on maintenance haemodialysis.
2. Assess iron stores every two months in dialysis patients. Serum ferritin is the most appropriate investigation (often TIBC is low). Replace with oral iron; use parenteral iron only if the oral iron is not absorbed.
3. Blood transfusion:
   a. In chronic renal failure (CRF):
      Generally the low Hb is well tolerated by patients with CRF. The beneficial effect of blood transfusion is short lived and it should be reserved for those patients with severe symptoms of anaemia. Do not attempt to raise the Hb to normal levels — this will suppress bone marrow production, and reduce the renal plasma flow which will further reduce the glomerular filtration rate
   b. In acute renal failure (ARF):
      A reasonable policy with ARF is to maintain the Hb at or above 10 g/dl with small transfusions of packed cells.
4. Androgen therapy (to stimulate erythropoiesis). This is *not* recommended as it is frequently unsuccessful and is associated with virilisation and cholestatic jaundice.

RED CELL CHANGES IN RENAL DISEASE

Blood film
RBC usually normochromic and normocytic, but anisopoikilocytosis, burr cells, occasional tear drop cells may be seen. Red cell fragments are seen in malignant hypertension, haemolytic-uraemic syndrome, and other causes of microangiopathic haemolytic anaemia (p. 243).

Polycythaemia
Due to increased, autonomous erythropoietin production by the kidneys. Rare, but can be seen with single or multiple renal cysts, hydronephrosis, renal tumours (particularly carcinoma), and after transplantation.

WHITE CELL CHANGES IN RENAL DISEASE

1. Neutrophilia (renal tract infection).
2. Neutropenia (renal failure, azathioprine therapy, hypersplenism).
3. Increased susceptibility to infection due to:
   a. Leucopenia
   b. Reduced chemotactic ability (acidosis)
   c. Reduced immunoglobulin synthesis (protein-calorie malnutrition)
   d. Immunosuppressive drugs (for auto-immune renal disease or transplant)
   e. Low complement (activated on dialysis tubing).

PLATELET AND COAGULATION FACTOR CHANGES IN RENAL DISEASE

Abnormalities seen

1. Thrombocytosis (renal infection, haematuria).
2. Thrombocytopenia. Rarely severe (hypersplenism, bone marrow suppression by toxic retention compounds, loss on dialysis tubing).
3. Abnormal platelet function.
4. Reduced levels of factors II, VII, IX and X (hepatorenal syndrome, vitamin K deficiency due to poor diet, antibiotic therapy, uraemic enteritis).
5. Disseminated intravascular coagulation (causes, and can be caused by, acute renal failure; also seen in acute graft rejection).
6. Nephrotic syndrome: urinary loss of factor IX and antithrombin III (AT III).
7. Abnormal factor VIII function.

Clinical manifestations

1. Bleeding tendency:
   a. Purpura is common
   b. Increased incidence of overt haemorrhage.
2. Thrombotic tendency:
   a. May be seen in patients undergoing haemodialysis (platelets are activated in the extra-corporeal circulation)
   b. Acquired AT III deficiency (nephrotic syndrome).

Investigations

1. PT, APTT, TT, (p. 173).
2. Platelet count.
3. Bleeding time.
4. Platelet aggregometry (if available).
5. With thrombosis, measurement of AT III level.

Unfortunately the results of these investigations correlate poorly with clinical severity of bleeding/thrombosis.

Treatment

Bleeding tendency (uncommon in patients on regular dialysis)

1. Avoid aspirin and other non-steroidal anti-inflammatory drugs.
2. Some patients may respond to cryoprecipitate and/or vitamin K.
3. Platelet concentrate is not helpful — the transfused platelets acquire the uraemic defect within hours.

Thrombotic tendency

1. In proven AT III deficiency prevent thrombosis with oral anti-coagulants. Established thrombosis should be treated with heparin and AT III concentrates (obtain advice from a specialist centre).
2. Patients on regular haemodialysis: the role of prophylactic anti-platelet agents (p. 187) has yet to be established.

REFERENCES

Desforges J F 1970 Anaemia in uraemia. Archives of Internal Medicine 126: 808–811
Erslev A J 1970 Anaemia of chronic renal disease. Archives of Internal Medicine 126: 774–780
Mansell M, Grimes A J 1979 Red and white cell abnormalities in chronic renal failure. British Journal of Haematology 42(2): 808–811

35. DRUG INDUCED HAEMATOLOGICAL DISEASE

The list of drugs that can cause haematological abnormalities is vast and only those most commonly implicated are mentioned here.

PATHOPHYSIOLOGICAL CLASSIFICATION OF ADVERSE DRUG EFFECTS

1. Predictable effect related to the known pharmacological action and dependent on the total dose of drug, e.g. marrow suppression due to methotrexate.
2. Unpredictable effect
   a. Hypersensitivity reaction, unrelated to pharmacological action but conditioned by previous exposure to the drug
   b. Idiosyncrasy. Adverse effect unrelated to the known pharmacological action and often occurring with the first dose given
   c. Often inevitable adverse effect, usually related to the known pharmacological action but dependent on a genetically determined metabolic abnormality in the patient, e.g. haemolysis due to primaquine in G6PD-deficiency.

ASSOCIATING THE DRUG WITH THE ADVERSE REACTION

This is often very difficult and requires a very careful history. Laboratory proof that a particular drug is responsible is usually not obtainable and a particular drug must often be withdrawn from the patient on clinical suspicion alone.

Diagnostic pointers

1. The drug involved has a known association with the particular adverse effect.
2. The pattern of clinical association, i.e. timing of reaction.

3. Simultaneous manifestations of drug sensitivity, e.g. jaundice, arthralgia, fever, rash, lupus syndrome.
4. Absence of other causes of the haematological abnormality.

Points to note in history

1. Length of exposure to drug (e.g. short exposure suggests hypersensitivity; long exposure typical of methyldopa auto-immune haemolysis).
2. Dose used (e.g. the higher the dose of methotrexate used, the greater the chance of marrow suppression).
3. Previous exposure to the drug.
4. Route of administration (e.g. aplasia due to chloramphenicol has been reported even after intra-ocular use).
5. Family history (e.g. familial increase in incidence of adverse reactions to chloramphenicol).
6. Detailed history of other drugs used (e.g. cross-reactivity shown with penicillins and cephalosporins in causing auto-immune haemolysis; similarly quinidine and quinine-induced thrombocytopenia).
7. Ethnic origin (e.g. severity of G6PD deficiency).
8. History of atopy (atopic individuals have an increased incidence of hypersensitivity to drugs).

Once suspicion strong that a particular drug has caused a particular adverse reaction:

1. If a serious reaction, or one not commonly associated with that particular drug report to the Committee on Safety of Medicines ('yellow card').
2. Warn the patient. It may be useful to give them a card to carry.

TYPES OF REACTION AND TREATMENT

The first line of treatment in all cases is to discontinue the drug thought to be responsible

Drug induced immune haemolysis

Methyldopa type haemolysis

Action
Exact mechanism not established but the drug provokes production of antibodies that have red-cell specificity (often directed against one of the Rhesus antigens) and the antibodies will react with normal red cells carrying that antigen even in the absence of the drug.

Clinical features
1. Usually develops after weeks or months of standard dose treatment.
2. Gradual onset of anaemia with mild jaundice and occasionally minimal splenomegaly.
3. Low haemoglobin, high reticulocyte count.
4. Blood film shows polychromasia and spherocytes.
5. DAT (Direct Antiglobulin Test = Direct Coomb's Test) positive and IAT (Indirect Antiglobulin Test = Indirect Coomb's Test) positive with and without drug present. The red cells are coated with IgG only.
6. Non-specific signs of haemolysis, urine urobilinogen present, raised serum bilirubin and HBDH.
   Haemolysis is predominantly extravascular.

Drug absorption immune haemolysis

Action
Drug-induced antibody has specificity for drug-related antigens that have become absorbed onto the red cell membrane. The red cells are coated with the drug during its administration and the anti-drug antibodies attach to the red cell which is then removed by the reticulo-endothelial system.

Causative drugs
1. High-dose penicillin (usually more than 10 mega units daily).
2. Normal dose cephalosporins.

Clinical and laboratory features
1. Rapid onset of haemolytic anaemia usually occurring one to two weeks after starting treatment.
2. Laboratory features as for methyldopa haemolysis except that:
   a. Spherocytes are not a marked feature
   b. IAT is positive in the presence of the drug but negative in its absence.

Immune-complex immune haemolysis

Action
Drug-induced antibody has specificity for the drug itself and the resulting drug/anti-drug-antibody immune-complex is adsorbed passively onto red cells. Complement is then activated and intravascular red cell lysis will ensue.

Causative drugs
Quinidine, phenacetin.

Clinical features
1. Often history of previous exposure to the drug.
2. Very abrupt onset of intravascular haemolysis within days of starting treatment.
3. Profound anaemia, brown urine, red-brown plasma, acute renal failure.

Laboratory features
1. Haemoglobin may be as low as 2–4 g/dl.
2. High reticulocyte count, often > 30%.
3. Spherocytes on blood film.
4. Free Hb in plasma, haemoglobinuria, haemosiderinuria, plus other non-specific features of haemolysis.
5. DAT positive, IAT positive in presence of drug, negative without drug. Usually complement only can be found on the red cell surface.

Treatment of drug-induced immune haemolysis
1. Stop the drug and do not reintroduce.
2. Prevention. Monitor haemoglobin every three months for a year in patients starting on methyldopa or when the dose is increased.
3. Role of blood transfusion. No place for it in stable mild anaemia i.e. Hb > 8 g/dl unless the patient has worrying symptoms, e.g. angina. Because of the positive indirect antiglobulin test, cross-matching blood for these patients is very difficult as all units of blood will appear to be incompatible. The incompatible reactions cannot be ignored, however, as they may be hiding a true transfusion allo-antibody reaction and transfusion may result in intravascular haemolysis of the units of blood involved thereby worsening the situation. However, in severe symptomatic anaemia, cautious transfusion of small quantities of blood (one or two units) may be necessary.
4. With profound intravascular haemolysis, usual measures for the treatment of incipient or established acute renal failure should be instituted.
5. Usually there is prompt reversal of haemolysis in the one to two weeks following withdrawal of the drug responsible. If there is no response in this time and the patient remains severely anaemic, oral corticosteroids (e.g. prednisolone at a dose of 40 mg/m^2/day) should be considered. Their use is debatable.

Other drugs known to cause immune haemolysis
Stibophen, quinine, PAS, chlorpromazine, fenfluramine, isoniazid, many sulpha drugs, ibuprofen.

Drug induced, non-immune, oxidative haemolysis

Action
The red cell is susceptible to oxidant stress which can cause changes in the haemoglobin molecule and in the red cell membrane leading to rigidity and lysis.

Oxidative damage usually occurs when there is an underlying abnormality of RBC metabolism rendering the cell more susceptible to oxidant stress. By far the most common cause is G6PD deficiency but other rare enzyme defects or unstable haemoglobins may be responsible. In rare cases a massive overdose of an oxidative chemical or drug may cause haemolysis in normal individuals. Babies may be particularly susceptible.

Causative drugs
1. Antimalarials: primaquine, chloroquine, mepacrine.
2. Sulpha derivatives: co-trimoxazole, sulphasalazine, dapsone.
3. Other antibiotics: penicillin, streptomycin, nitrofurantoin, isoniazid, PAS.
4. Anti-helminthics: stibophane.
5. Others: phenylhydrazine, quinidine, probenecid, aspirin.

Clinical features
Typically symptoms start three days after taking the drug, with jaundice, anaemia and haemoglobinuria.
Three different clinical syndromes:
1. Methaemoglobinaemia with chronic intravascular haemolysis. Most commonly seen with dapsone, sulphasalazine, phenacetin.
2. Acute intravascular haemolysis ± methaemoglobinaemia. Typical with G6PD deficiency and oxidant drugs or fava beans.
3. Acute intravascular haemolysis, methaemoglobinaemia, disseminated intravascular coagulation, acute renal failure. Rare. Seen with accidental or deliberate massive overdoses of oxidant agent, e.g. chlorate weed killer, arsine gas.

Laboratory features
1. Low red cell G6PD (p. 38).
2. Blood film shows fragmented red cells: Heinz bodies may be seen with supravital staining.
3. Methaemoglobinaemia.
4. Haemoglobin and haemosiderin in urine.
5. All other non-specific signs of haemolysis (p. 30)

Treatment
1. Usually no specific treatment is needed as the haemolysis rapidly settles once the drug is withdrawn. Often the haemolysis is self-limiting providing drug dosage is not increased as reticulocytes contain high levels of G6PD and resist haemolysis.
2. Preventative: screen for G6PD deficiency in childhood and test families of deficient patients, and warn them which drugs not to take.
   The clinical necessity of using an oxidant drug may outweigh the risk of inducing haemolysis in some situations e.g. treatment of malaria with proguanil or chloroquine does not usually induce worrying haemolysis though drug resistant parasites may require the use of more oxidant drugs.
3. In severe intravascular haemolysis, blood transfusion will be necessary. Careful monitoring of renal function, platelet count and coagulation should be carried out and the complications of renal failure and DIC treated appropriately.

Drug induced aplastic anaemia

Action

1. Dose-related reversible marrow suppression affecting mainly the red cell series but sometimes also white cells and platelets.
2. A more severe, probably idiosyncratic suppression of all cell lines in the bone marrow.

Causative drugs

1. Chloramphenicol: approximate risk of severe aplasia 1 in 20 000.
2. Anti-inflammatory drugs: phenylbutazone, oxyphenbutazone, indomethacin: commoner in the elderly and usually only after months of treatment, approximate risk of severe aplasia 1 in 500 000.
3. Gold (sodium aurothiomalate): usually dose-dependent but in a small group of patients the aplasia is an idiosyncratic reaction appearing early in treatment.
4. Others: co-trimoxazole, phenytoin, allopurinol.

Clinical and laboratory features

1. Aplastic anaemia is the most serious of the drug-induced haematological disorders with a very significant morbidity and mortality.
2. Very variable severity and time-relationship.
3. Variable pancytopenia with low reticulocyte count.
4. Bone marrow trephine shows aplasia sometimes with small areas of normal, or even increased cellularity.
5. Raised HbF level.

Treatment

1. Usually, withdrawal of the offending drug does not result in rapid improvement of the blood count. The clinical outlook is similar to that in idiopathic aplastic anaemia, the management of which is dealt with in Chapter
2. If recovery occurs warn patient about the drug (and its chemical relatives).

Drug induced agranulocytosis

Action

1. Direct toxic damage to neutrophil precursors.
2. Immune mediated (suppression of granulopoiesis, destruction of mature granulocytes or auto-antibody production with white-cell specificity).

Causative drugs

1. Sulpha drugs: co-trimoxazole.
2. Anti-thyroid: propylthiouracil, carbimazole.
3. Others: phenothiazines, penicillin.

Clinical features

1. Idiosyncratic unpredictable response. Usually occurs one to two weeks after first exposure or immediately after re-exposure. Constitutional symptoms, e.g. fever, arthralgia, chills, common, as is oral ulceration.
2. Dose-related, insidious reaction often after weeks of treatment. Present with bacterial infection, occasionally overwhelming. Prodromal constitutional symptoms unusual.

Laboratory features

1. Severe granulocytopenia, neutrophils $< 0.2 \times 10^9/1$.
2. Haemoglobin and platelets normal.
3. Marrow findings variable but useful to exclude neutropenia due to megaloblastosis.
4. Exclude SLE and infectious mononucleosis with Paul-Bunnell test and anti-nuclear factor.
5. Special tests for CFU-C assays, leukoagglutinins can be arranged with specialist laboratories but they are often inconclusive.

Treatment

The prognosis is good providing the patient can be tided over the period of agranulocytosis (see Chapters 12 and 15 for management).

Drug induced thrombocytopenia

Action

1. Increased destruction of platelets in peripheral blood. Usually immune mediated, e.g. quinine, digoxin.
2. Direct toxic effect on marrow megakaryocytes resulting in reduced platelet production, e.g. thiazides.

Causative drugs

Co-trimoxazole, quinidine, quinine, phenylbutazone, oxyphenbutazone indomethacin, frusemide, thiazides, chloramphenicol, rifampicin, sodium aurothiomalate.

Clinical features

1. Commonly abrupt onset of purpura developing over hours. May be accompanied by constitutional symptoms.
2. Often occurs within days of last dose of course of drug lasting for days or weeks. With gold-induced thrombocytopenia, the delay between the last dose given and symptoms developing may be months.
3. Any haemorrhagic manifestation is possible but oral haemorrhagic bullae, petechiae, gum bleeding and haematuria are probably the most common. Deep tissue bleeds and haemarthroses are unusual.

Laboratory features
1. Platelet count reduced, often lower than $20 \times 10^9/1$.
2. Rest of blood count normal unless the bleeding has resulted in anaemia.
3. Bone marrow aspiration may show normal, decreased or increased megakaryocytes with variable platelet budding. The morphology depends on the mechanism of the thrombocytopenia.
4. Usually the haemorrhagic manifestations will subside within 24 hours of withdrawal of the drug and the platelet count will recover to normal over the next one to two weeks.

Treatment
1. Stop the drug.
2. Replace significant blood loss with blood transfusion. If bleeding manifestations are prominent take measures to prevent cerebral haemorrhage by preventing episodes of raised intracranial pressure, i.e. bed rest, treat hypertension.
3. Avoid drugs e.g. aspirin, anti-inflammatory agents, that affect platelet function.
4. Because the thrombocytopenia is often immune-mediated, platelet transfusions are usually useless as a prophylactic measure as the transfused platelets are so rapidly destroyed, though they may be used in desperation for life-threatening bleeds.
5. If gold is the drug thought to be responsible, treat with the chelating agent dimercaprol.
6. If recovery is slow and bleeding severe, consider using oral corticosteroids e.g. prednisolone at a dose of 20–40 mg/m²/day.

Drug induced megaloblastic anaemia

Action
1. Disturbance of B12 metabolism.
2. Disturbance of folic acid metabolism.
3. Inhibition of DNA synthesis unrelated to B12 or folic acid metabolism.

Causative drugs
1. Anti-folate: oral contraceptives, anti-convulsants (diphenylhydantoin, primidone, barbiturates), cycloserine, trimethoprim, triamterene, pyrimethamine, methotrexate.
2. Anti-B12: metformin, PAS, neomycin, colchicine, slow release potassium, nitrous oxide.
3. DNA inhibitors: hydroxyurea, azathioprine, 6-mercaptopurine, 5-fluorouracil, 6-thioguanine.

Clinical features
Insidious onset of anaemia with associated megaloblastic clinical features (see Ch. 3 on macrocytic anaemia).

Laboratory features
Identical to those in megaloblastic anaemia due to other causes (see Ch. 3 on macrocytic anaemia).

Treatment
1. Withdraw drug if possible.
2. Treat with replacement i.m. hydroxocobalamin (neo-cytamen) 1 mg for at least six doses, (the frequency determined by the severity of anaemia) and/or replacement with folic acid 5 mg oral t.d.s. either for three months after drug stopped or permanently if drug continued.
   There is no evidence that treating anti-convulsant-induced folate deficiency with folic acid increases the incidence of fits.

Drug induced sideroblastic anaemia

Action
Interference with the metabolism of erythroblast mitochondria.

Causative drugs
Chloramphenicol, alcohol, lead, isoniazid, cycloserine, pyrazinamide.

Clinical and laboratory features
1. Non-specific features of slowly evolving anaemia.
2. Haemoglobin rarely less than 8 g/dl.
3. Red cells hypochromic, sometimes microcytic, occasionally macrocytic or dimorphic.
4. Punctate basophilia in red cells.
5. Reticulocytes 1–4%.
6. Serum iron raised, TIBC reduced.
7. Bone marrow aspirate shows vast accumulation of reticuloendothelial iron and ringed sideroblasts.

Treatment
1. Once drug is stopped, try pyridoxine 100–500 mg orally daily and folic acid 5 mg t.d.s.
2. If no response to pyridoxine and folate and patient remains symptomatically anaemic, blood transfusion may be necessary.

REFERENCES

Dawson A A 1979 Drug-induced haematological disease. British Medical Journal 1: 1195–1197
Gordon-Smith E C (ed) 1980 Haematological effects of drug therapy. Clinics in Haematology 9(3)

Part 9
LABORATORY
FINDINGS

36. BLOOD FILM ABNORMALITIES

RED CELL MORPHOLOGICAL ABNORMALITIES

Red cell size

An experienced microscopist may appreciate significant degrees of microcytosis (small red cells) and macrocytosis (large red cells) from examination of the blood film. However, the majority of modern blood counters provide a more sensitive index of variation in cell volume than can be appreciated by eye.

Anisocytosis
Variation in cell size. A fairly non-specific abnormality seen in the blood of many ill people. It is particularly noticeable after recent treatment of a haematinic deficiency or blood transfusion. Many cell counting machines produce an electronic index of anisocytosis, the RDW (Red cell size, Distribution Width).

Red cell shape

Poikilocytosis
Variation in cell shape. Like anisocytosis, minor degrees are commonly seen in the blood of ill persons. Certain varieties of poikilocytosis (shapes of red cell) have particular clinical significance:

1. Burr cells (red cells having regular spiky projections) are characteristic of renal failure.
2. Schistocytes (red cell fragments of variable shape), helmet cells and fragmented cells frequently occur together and usually indicate damage to the red cell by fibrin strands in small blood vessels — a microangiopathic blood picture. Common causes are disseminated intravascular coagulation, vasculitis, glomerulonephritis and thrombotic thrombocytopenic purpura. Fragmented cells may also be seen in the blood as a result of trauma by blood turbulence associated with tight stenosis of heart valves and artificial heart valves.

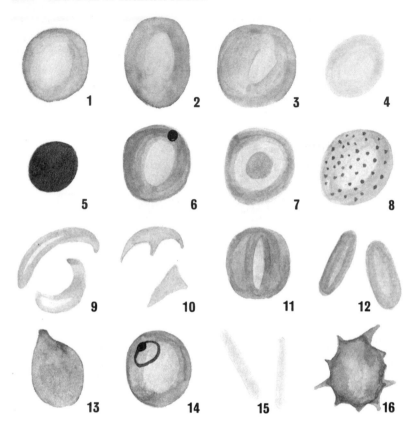

Figs 36.1–36.16 Red cell morphological abnormalities. 1 Normal red cell. 2 Oval macrocyte (megaloblastic change). 3 Round macrocyte (liver disease, hypothyroidism). 4 Hypochromic microcyte. 5 Spherocyte. 6 Howell-Jolly body. 7 Target cell. 8 Basophilic stippling. 9 Sickle cells. 10 Fragmented cells. 11 Stomatocyte. 12 Elliptocytes. 13 Tear-drop poikilocyte. 14 Malarial ring trophozoite. 15 Pencil cells (seen in iron deficiency). 16 Burr cell

3. Acanthocytes (red cells with multiple irregular sharp spiny projections) are seen in abetalipoproteinaemia, alcoholic liver disease, and in small numbers after splenectomy.

4. Target cells have too much membrane for the contents of the cell and are characterised by a dark staining centre (surrounded by a pale ring and then a dark staining peripheral ring) rather than the usual pale centre. They are seen in liver disease (commonly with slight macrocytosis) iron deficiency (with hypochromia and microcytosis) the thalassaemias and haemoglobinopathies and after splenectomy (with Howell-Jolly bodies and spherocytes).

5. Tear-drop cells (pear-shaped cells) are characteristic of myelofibrosis, accompanying the leucoerythroblastic blood picture commonly seen in this condition.

6. Spherocytes are cells that have lost their usual biconcave disc shape and are spherical. They may be seen in the blood in any case of haemolysis, but are particularly common in hereditary spherocytosis and haemolytic jaundice of the newborn due to ABO antibodies. Other common causes are autoimmune haemolytic anaemia and post splenectomy (when Howell-Jolly bodies and target cells are also seen).

Red cell staining

1. *Hypochromia*: pale staining of red cells due to low haemoglobin content (usually occurs with microcytosis). The blood count will show a low MCH (mean corpuscular haemoglobin). Seen in iron deficiency, the thalassaemias, sideroblastic anaemia and (occasionally) in the anaemia of chronic disease. Variation in depth of staining of red cells may sometimes suggest that two populations of red cells are present — one normally haemoglobinised and one hypochromic. This is termed a dimorphic picture and is commonly seen when a hypochromic anaemia is treated initially with haematinics or transfusion and also in sideroblastic anaemia.
2. *Polychromasia* refers to a grey-blue tint to the red cell in stained films and is a characteristic of young red cells. Polychromasia will usually accompany a high reticulocyte count and mild macrocytosis (young cells are big cells). This regenerative blood picture is seen in haemolysis and during recovery from bleeding. The reticulocyte count can only be assessed by a blood film stained by a special technique.

Red cell inclusions

The spleen is normally responsible for removing inclusions from red cells and increased numbers of all types of inclusions are seen after splenectomy and in hyposplenic states.

1. Howell-Jolly bodies which are nuclear remnants, the commonest red cell inclusion.
2. Pappenheimer bodies (iron containing granules) will be found in red cells which are then termed siderocytes. Siderocytes are also found in the blood in iron overload states.
3. Heinz bodies are particles of denatured protein (haemoglobin) stuck to the inside of the red cell membrane and require special stains for their demonstration. They are seen in conditions where the red cell has been exposed to chemical poisons. Common causes are G6PD deficiency after treatment with oxidant drugs, chemical poisoning, and the presence of an inherently unstable haemoglobin in the red cell.

4. Basophilic stippling is seen in a variety of anaemias, but classically following lead poisoning and in pyrimidine-5-nucleotidase deficiency.
5. Malarial parasites.

Abnormal arrangements of red cells

1. Rouleaux are regular branching chains of red cells seen in any cause of a high ESR (Ch. 37).
2. Cold agglutinates are haphazard irregular clumps of red cells caused by an antibody present in the patients serum which agglutinates the red cells when the blood sample cools below body temperature. The red cell agglutinates may be visible to the naked eye in the sample tube, and may cause a 'pseudomacrocytosis' in the blood count as the instrument counts clumps of red cells rather than single cells. The agglutinates are abolished by heating the blood to 37°C. The phenomenon may be confirmed by performing a cold agglutinin titre using serum removed from the patient's red cells whilst still at body temperature.

WHITE CELL MORPHOLOGICAL ABNORMALITIES

Leucocytosis (Ch. 9) and leucopenia (Ch. 12) may be appreciated from the blood film and the differential white cell count may reveal increases in specific white cell types.

1. Neutrophil left shift denotes the presence of immature neutrophils (stab cells or metamyelocytes) in the peripheral blood. The cells have been recruited into the blood from the bone marrow and spleen in response to stress, commonly infection or trauma. Usually a neutrophil leucocytosis is present. A more marked degree of neutrophil left shift is present if even earlier stages of white cell maturation (myelocytes, promyelocytes, blasts) are present in the peripheral blood. If nucleated red cells are also present then this is a leucoerythroblastic blood picture (see Ch. 5).
2. Neutrophil right shift is the presence of multilobed hypersegmented neutrophils in the blood, characteristic of megaloblastic anaemias
3. Toxic granulation describes the violet granules that may be seen in neutrophil cytoplasm in bacterial infections. Dohle bodies, rarely seen, have similar significance.
4. Reactive lymphocytes are seen in viral infections, particularly glandular fever. Turk cells are a particular variety of reactive lymphocyte, but are less specific to viral infections.

Platelet morphological abnormalities

An increased platelet count (thrombocytosis — Ch. 8) and reduced platelet count (thrombocytopenia — Ch. 11) may be readily appreciated from examination of the blood film.

1. Giant platelets are characteristically seen in the myeloproliferative diseases (chronic granulocytic leukaemia, myelofibrosis, essential thrombocythaemia, and polycythaemia rubra vera). Minor increases in platelet size are best appreciated by electronic measurement of the mean platelet volume (MPV) in the blood count.

2. Platelet clumping on the blood film commonly results from partial clotting of the blood sample due to difficult venepuncture, delay in transferring blood into the specimen bottle, or inadequate mixing. Some patients have platelets that clump whatever precautions are taken. This clumping of platelets may be the cause of a false low platelet count.

REFERENCES

Hayhoe F C J, Flemans R J 1982 A colour atlas of haematological cytology, 2nd edn. Wolfe Medical, London
O'Connor B H 1984 A colour atlas and instruction manual of peripheral blood cell morphology. Williams & Wilkins, Baltimore

37. ERYTHROCYTE SEDIMENTATION RATE (ESR)

DEFINITION

The speed of settling of the red cell layer of anticoagulated whole blood allowed to sediment in a vertical calibrated tube. It is usually measured after one hour.

CAUSES OF ELEVATED ESR

An elevated ESR is correlated with rouleaux formation in the blood, which in turn is related to high concentrations of fibrinogen, gamma globulin, and other acute phase proteins. The ESR is elevated in a multitude of disease processes including infections, malignancies, collagen and autoimmune diseases. Its value lies principally as a screening test in the detection of a disease process and in following the course of a diagnosed disease. The ESR rises with advancing years and is also mildly elevated by anaemia of any cause.

An ESR over 140mm/hour is unusual in diseases other than myeloma, Waldenstrom's disease, suppurative TB, and connective tissue disorders.

PLASMA VISCOSITY

May be used as a substitute for the ESR, being quicker to perform and not affected by red cell abnormalities. It reflects an increase in acute phase proteins in the plasma.

REFERENCE

Gibbs D 1982 Symptomless abnormalities — ESR. British Journal of Hospital Medicine May: 493–496

Part 10
APPENDIX

38. PRACTICAL PROCEDURES IN HAEMATOLOGY

Use a clean no-touch technique for the following procedures. In neutropenic patients use gloves and a mask.

PUTTING UP A DRIP

Obtaining satisfactory access to the circulation is an important technique to learn in the management of haematology patients. Veins are these patients lifelines — do not destroy them.

Making the vein appear

1. Better to spend time finding a good vein than 'having a stab', demoralising the patient and causing a haematoma.
2. Apply a tourniquet to the upper arm, or alternatively use a blood pressure cuff inflated to halfway between systolic and diastolic pressures.
3. Clenching and unclenching the fist will assist in distending the veins.
4. Illuminate the skin using a bright oblique light — often the shape of a vein can be seen beneath the skin better than its colour. Veins are often better felt than seen.
5. If a satisfactory vein cannot be located, immerse the arm in hot water to dilate the veins.
6. Try to choose the most peripheral vein that can be easily cannulated.
7. Avoid areas over joints if possible, to allow mobility of the arm.
8. Do not leave the tourniquet on unnecessarily — it is uncomfortable and may cause purpura in thrombocytopenic patients.

Insertion of cannula

1. Select a suitable cannula. Large cannulae are more traumatic to the vein, but can sustain rapid infusion rates e.g. in haemorrhage, and are less easily blocked.

251

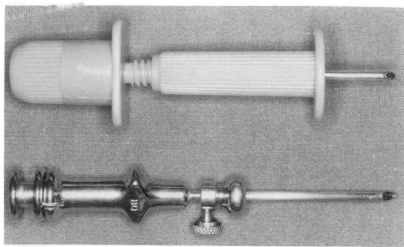

Fig. 38.1 Bone marrow aspirate needles. Disposable Klima needle (top) and Salah needle (bottom)

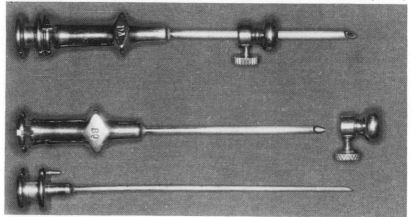

Fig. 38.2 Salah aspirate needle assembled for use (top) and disassembled (bottom).

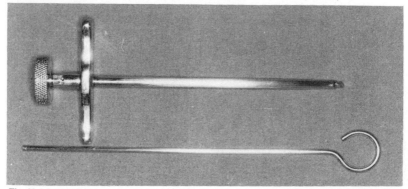

Fig. 38.3 Jamshidi biopsy needle assembled for use

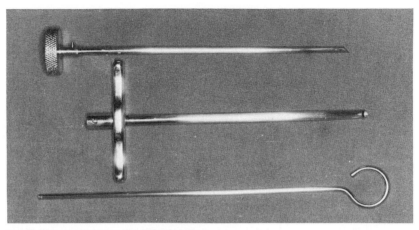

Fig. 38.4 Jamshidi biopsy needle disassembled

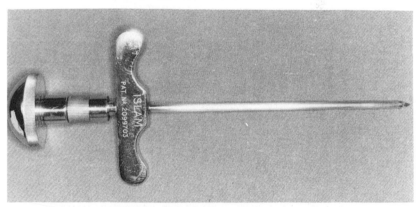

Fig. 38.5 Islam biopsy needle assembled for use

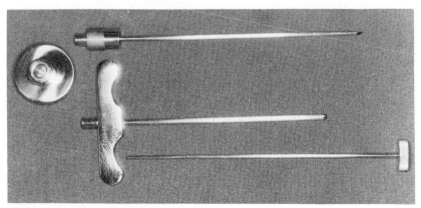

Fig. 38.6 Islam biopsy needle disassembled

2. Clean the skin with suitable antiseptic.
3. Using a 1 or 2 ml syringe inject a bleb of local anaesthetic e.g. 2% lignocaine, intradermally over the chosen site for insertion.
4. Wait for anaesthetic to work — minimum 1 minute.
5. Insert the cannula and needle through the bleb of local anaesthetic into the vein. Entry into the vein will be shown by 'flashback' of blood into the hub of the cannula. Partly withdraw the needle to sheath the point, and advance the cannula into the vein.
6. Release the cuff, to prevent a spill of blood, and remove the needle from the cannula.
7. Connect the drip, or a syringe if blood is being taken. (Once drip fluid has been infused the drip cannula should not be used to take blood samples, as it will be contaminated by infusion fluid.)
8. Cover and protect the drip site.

EXCHANGE TRANSFUSION IN ADULTS

There are a variety of methods for exchange transfusion in adults, many of which are satisfactory, but we consider the following method to be optimal:

1. Set up a drip in one arm (see above) and start transfusing first unit of blood.
2. Insert a large (16 gauge) butterfly into the antecubital vein of the other arm and a resealable rubber cap into its hub. Use a standard venesection bag to take blood, inserting the needle through the rubber reseal bung.
3. When the bag is full, remove the blood pack needle from the rubber bung. As this is a large needle, it may be necessary to replace the rubber bung if it leaks. Fill the butterfly with heparin rinse (e.g. 500 units of heparin in 2 ml of saline for injection) to prevent it clotting when not in use.
4. Match rate of venesection with rate of infusion.
5. If blood flow is slow on the venesection arm insert a three-way tap between the butterfly hub and reseal bung and use a syringe to alternately draw blood from the vein and eject it into the bag.

BONE MARROW EXAMINATION

Sites

1. Posterior iliac crest: suitable for both aspirate and biopsy. The site of choice for marrow examination except in obese patients when the anatomy may be obscured.
2. Anterior iliac crest: suitable for both aspirate and biopsy. The bone tends to be harder than at the posterior iliac crest.

3. Sternum: easy access for aspirate, but not suitable for biopsy. Some patients may find the anterior chest approach alarming, ad there is a risk of perforating the sternum with damage to great vessels. The needle guard must be correctly adjusted.

Aspirate procedure (posterior iliac crest)

1. Fully explain the procedure to the patient.
2. Position patient on side or prone. Locate the posterior superior iliac spine by palpation (Figs 38.7, 38.8).
3. Clean the skin with iodine solution (ask about allergy).
4. Infiltrate the skin with local anaesthetic e.g. 2% lignocaine and then inject the subcutaneous tissues and (most importantly) the periosteum.
5. Wait for anaesthetic to work. Test for anaesthesia using a venepuncture needle.
6. Check that the syringe fits on the marrow aspirate needle. The guard need not be used when aspirating from the posterior iliac crest site.

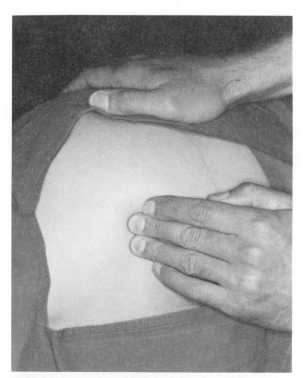

Fig. 38.7 Locating superior posterior iliac spine by palpation

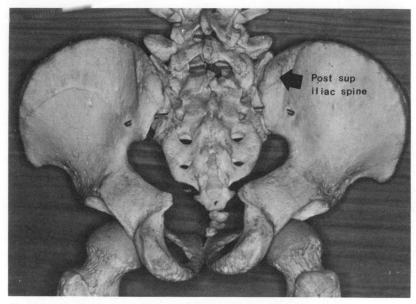

Post sup
iliac spine

Fig. 38.8 Position of posterior superior iliac spine

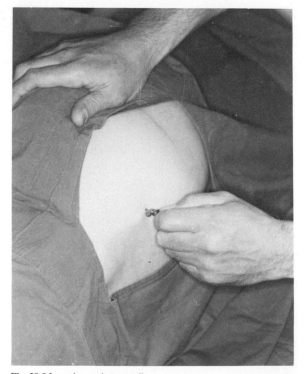

Fig. 38.9 Inserting aspirate needle

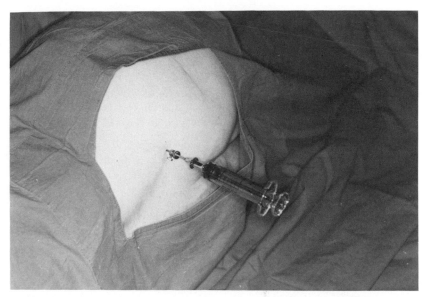

Fig. 38.10 Syringe attached to aspirate needle

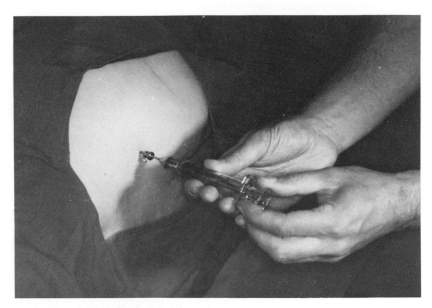

Fig. 38.11 Aspiration of marrow

7. Using a rotational oscillatory motion (similar to that of a ratchet screwdriver) penetrate the cortex to a depth of approximately 1 cm. A sudden loss of resistance may be felt as the cortex is penetrated (Fig. 38.9).

8. Remove the stilette, attach a 10 ml syringe, and gently aspirate 0.5 ml of marrow (Figs 38.10, 38.11). Warn the patient to expect the short, sharp pain of suction. If a dry tap see below.

9. Partially replace stilette to stem blood flow. More marrow may be aspirated with a second syringe if required for further investigations.

10. Make marrow slides (see below).

11. Remove needle and apply a dressing.

Dry tap

In the event of no marrow appearing in the syringe on aspiration:

1. Fully replace stilette, rotate needle slightly, and try again. If still dry:

2. Using a fresh needle, (clotting factors will have been activated by now) try again in a slightly different direction, using a 30 or 50 ml syringe. If still dry, take a biopsy (see below).

Trephine marrow biopsy

Indications

1. Dry tap on aspirate.

2. Suspected secondary carcinoma or lymphoma.

3. Suspected myelofibrosis or aplastic anaemia.

4. In other situations a biopsy may give additional information, but is a more difficult and uncomfortable procedure than aspirate.

Procedure

1. Clean the skin and anaesthetise the posterior iliac crest as described for marrow aspirate.

2. Very nervous patients may benefit from sedation, and oral or i.v. analgesia may be used. In children the antihistamine type of sedatives are unsatisfactory for bone marrows. Ideally use ketamine 1–2 mg/kg i.v. over 5 minutes to induce a short period of general anaesthesia. The child should not have eaten for 4 hours, and full resuscitation facilities should be available with a paediatrician/anaesthetist present.

3. Insert the biopsy needle in the same fashion as an aspirate needle (see above) to a depth of approximately 0.5 cm into the cortex, so that it supports its own weight (Figs 38.12 and 38.13).

4. Remove the stilette (Fig. 38.14).

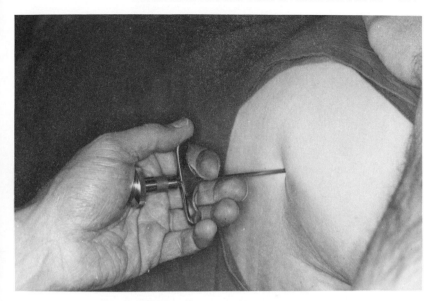

Fig. 38.12 Biopsy needle is inserted into right posterior iliac crest

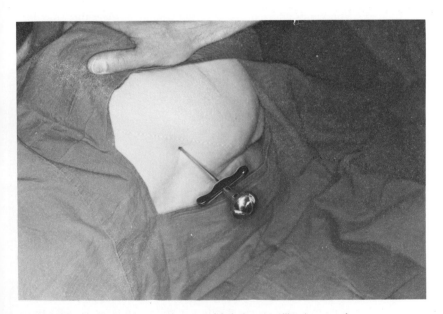

Fig. 38.13 The needle should support its own weight before the stillete is removed

5. Advance the needle slowly but firmly using the same oscillatory motion 1–3 cm, aiming for the anterior superior iliac spine. A core of bone marrow should now have entered the tip of the biopsy needle (Fig. 38.15).

6. This core must now be broken off by rapidly rotating the needle two revolutions clockwise, then two counter-clockwise. Also, advance the needle slightly (< 0.5 cm) aiming in a slightly different direction.

7. Slowly and cautiously withdraw the needle ensuring that the skin does not 'tent' as the needle leaves the cortex, as this may suck out the biopsy into the subcutaneous tissue.

8. Have an assistant apply pressure to the wound to ensure haemostasis.

9. Push out the biopsy using the blunt pusher provided with the biopsy needle, always inserting it into the needle at the sharp end, never the hub end (the biopsy needle tapers to its tip, and pushing the biopsy out the wrong way may crush it) (Fig. 38.16).

10. Deposit the biopsy on a slide, and then transfer it to histological fixative. The slide may be stained (a 'touch prep.') if the aspirate has been a dry tap.

11. Apply a pressure dressing to the wound. Inspect this later for evidence of bleeding in thrombocytopenic patients.

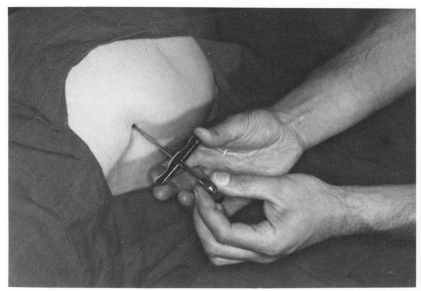

Fig. 38.14 Removing stillete

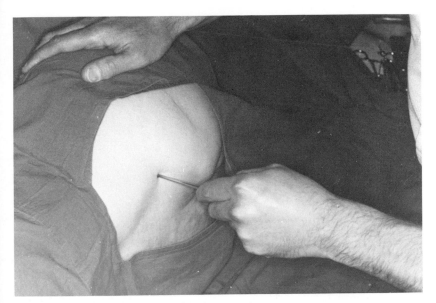

Fig. 38.15 Advancing needle a further 1–3 cm

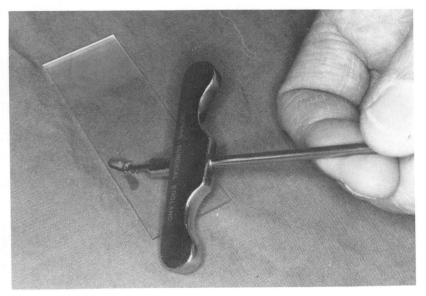

Fig. 38.16 Pushing out the biopsy onto a slide

Making marrow films

The same method is used for blood and bone marrow. When using fresh (unanticoagulated) material speed is essential to make the smears before clotting occurs.

1. Place a drop of marrow at one end of the slide (Fig. 38.17).
2. Apply the edge of another slide to the surface of the opposite end of this slide (Fig. 38. 18).
3. Pressing down, with the slides at 45 degrees to each other, back the top slide into the drop of marrow, so that it spreads along its edge (Fig. 38.19).
4. Reverse the direction of the top slide, spreading the marrow film (Fig. 38.20).

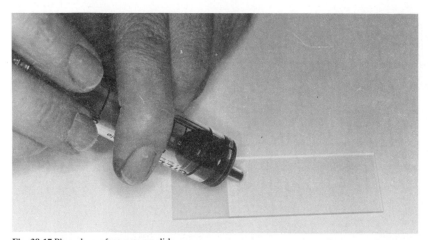

Fig. 38.17 Place drop of marrow on slide

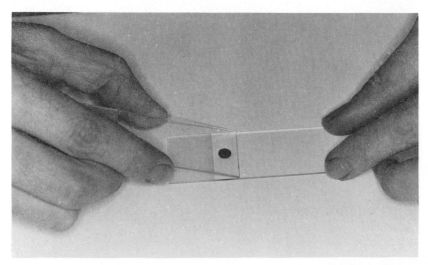

Fig. 38.18 Apply second slide as shown

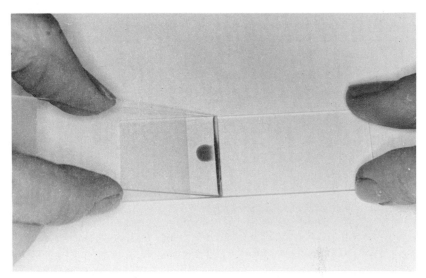

Fig. 38.19 Back top slide into marrow and spread

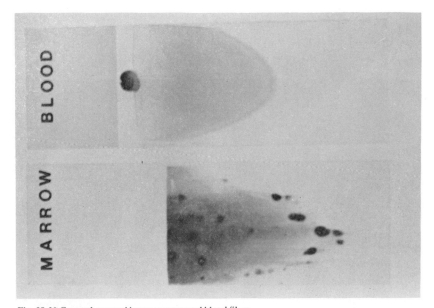

Fig. 38.20 Correctly spread bone marrow and blood films

CENTRAL VENOUS CATHETERS (HICKMAN)

These wide lumen silicone rubber catheters may be used for the administration of all intravenous solutions and the drawing of blood samples. Consider their use in all patients commencing intensive induction chemotherapy or marrow transplantation

Insertion

1. Insertion of these catheters is generally performed in theatre by a surgeon.
2. The catheter is threaded into the subclavian vein through a incision beneath the clavicle.
3. The other end of the catheter is then tunnelled subcutaneously to an exit on the anterior chest wall. This subcutaneous course reduces the risk of skin organisms gaining access to the circulation.
4. The position of the catheter is checked by a CXR (Fig. 38.21).
5. The catheter is held in place by a stitch at its exit point and by the formation of fibrous tissue around a special cuff lying in the subcutaneous tissue close to the exit point.

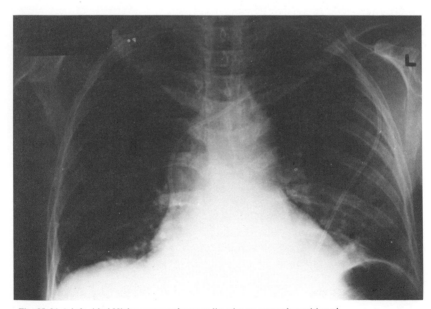

Fig. 38.21 A left-sided Hickman central venous line shown correctly positioned

Catheter care

All manipulations of the catheter are performed using strict aseptic technique with gloves and a mask. To prevent air embolism the catheter must be clamped with rubber sheathed forceps before each disconnection.

Heparin lock
1. In use the catheter should be flushed through with heparinised saline at every disconnection or at least once daily.
2. When not in continuous use the catheter may be 'capped off' using the sterile plug provided after filling the catheter with 2 ml of 1 in 1000 heparin. This heparin lock should be replaced at least twice weekly.

Blocked catheters
1. Attempt to flush the catheter with 2 ml of heparin rinse. Do not use force.
2. Connect a 20 ml syringe of normal saline and attempt to aspirate from the catheter.
   If unsuccessful:
3. Inject 1 ml of streptokinase (10 000–20 000 units), clamp the catheter and leave for at least one hour. Then attempt aspiration as above.

Catheter removal

1. Clamp and disconnect the catheter.
2. Clean the exit site and area round it with antiseptic.
3. Infiltrate the skin and subcutaneous tissue around the cuff with 2% lignocaine.
4. Make 1 cm incision over the cuff.
5. Free the cuffed segment of catheter by blunt dissection.
6. Remove the catheter by applying cautious traction.
7. Apply pressure to the area for a few minutes to effect haemostasis.
8. Suture the wound and apply a dressing.

39. NORMAL VALUES AND CORRECT SAMPLES

The following are guidelines only — consult with your laboratory as local ranges may vary with the methods of assay. This is particularly relevant with haematinic assays.

Measurement	Range	Units	Sample
Red cell count	M 4.5–6.5 F 3.8–5.8	$\times 10^{12}/1$ $\times 10^{12}/1$	EDTA (sequestrene)
Haemoglobin	M 13.0–18.0 F 11.5–16.5	g/dl g/dl	EDTA (sequestrene)
PCV	M 0.4–0.5 F 0.35–0.47	ratio ratio	EDTA (sequestrene)
MCV	78–96	fl.	EDTA (sequestrene)
MCH	27–32	pg.	EDTA (sequestrene)
MCHC	30–34	g/dl	EDTA (sequestrene)
Reticulocytes absolute count	0.2–2.0 10–100	% $10^9/1$	EDTA (sequestrene)
Total WBC	3.5–11.0	$10^9/1$	EDTA (sequestrene)

Differential WBC count:
  Neutrophils
  Lymphocytes
  Monocytes
  Eosinophils
  Basophils
	
	2.0–7.5
	1.5–4.0
	0.2–0.8
	< 0.4
	< 0.1
		
		$10^9/1$
		$10^9/1$
		$10^9/1$
		$10^9/1$
		$10^9/1$
			
			EDTA (sequestrene)
			EDTA (sequestrene)
			EDTA (sequestrene)
			EDTA (sequestrene)
			EDTA (sequestrene)

Platelet count	150–400	$10^9/1$	EDTA (sequestrene)
Red cell mass	M 25–35 F 20–30	ml/kg ml/kg	In vivo investigation
Plasma volume Total blood volume	40–50 60–80	ml/kg ml/kg	arrange with laboratory
Serum iron	12–32	mmol/l	Serum
TIBC	45–72	mmol/l	Serum
B12	150–900	ng/l	Serum
Serum folate	3–15	ng/l	Serum
RBC folate	160–640	ng/1	EDTA
ESR < 50 years ESR > 50 years	< 20 < 30	mm/hr mm/hr	Liquid citrate (1 in 5)

266

Measurement	Range	Units	Sample
Bleeding time (Template)	<9.5	mins	In vivo investigation
Prothrombin time	< 3 secs. over control		Liquid citrate
Prothrombin ratio	< 1.4		(1 in 10)
Activated partial thromboplastin time	< 7 secs. over control		Liquid citrate (1 in 10)
Thrombin time	< 3 secs. over control		Liquid citrate (1 in 10)
Fibrinogen	1.5–4.0	g/l	Liquid citrate (1 in 10)
Fibrinogen degradation products	< 10	μg/ml	Special sample tube

INDEX

269